2002

To: Claire

Peace + Joy fill your heart and when it is heavy, lift it with hope, faith, & love. Dare to dream... Rainbows ARE real! Thank you for your kind + comforting words over the years. You are such a lovely woman!

Fondly,
Barbara Dooling

Impossible Choices
The Lemonade Collection™

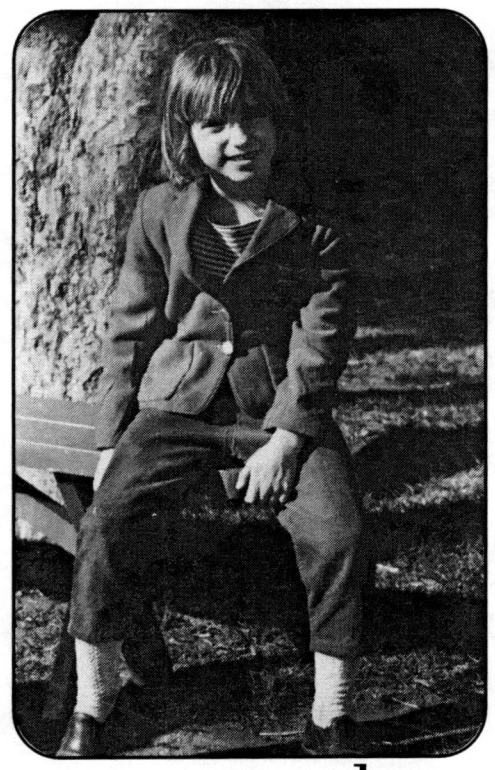

Barbara Dooling
Edited by Noreen Wise

HuckleberryPress.com
1-800-606-0541

Impossible Choices

A Huckleberry Press Book
The Lemonade Collection ™

Text Copyright ' 2002 by Barbara Dooling
Pictures Copyright ' 2002 byBarbara Dooling
All other Copyrights ' 2002 by Huckleberry Press

All rights reserved. No part of this book may be reproduced or utilized in any form by photostat, microfilm, xerography, electronic, or any other means, or incorporated into any information retrieval system, electronic or mechanical, without the written permission of the publisher.

All inquiries should be addressed to:
HuckleberryPress.com
P.O. Box 573
So. Glastonbury, CT 06073-0573
1-800-606-0541

Reading guides can be found at:
HuckleberryPress.com

Made in the United States
Publication Year 2001
10 9 8 7 6 5 4 3 2 1
ISBN 1-58584-522-1 • LCCN: 01-13070

Cover and graphic design by The Huckleberry Press creative team:
Lang Wethington, Noreen Wise

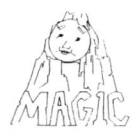

Three percent of the net revenues of all Huckleberry Press products
will be donated to the Magic Foundation.™

For Kara

*"He who remains cheerful in spirit
and sees only the good side of all things,
who never allows himself to be spiritually downcast
but keeps his head high and courage in his heart...
he sets in motion those fine, still powers,
which make every step through life easier for him."*

⁓Ralph Weld Trine

Acknowledgements

It is impossible to name everyone who has made a difference in getting me to this moment; such a list might be mistaken for the Boston white pages. The overflowing human kindness, good deeds, generosity, and loving cannot be bound. I am forever grateful to all of you, and owe more than the thanks that I can conjure up in a short passage of acknowledgments.

To my very special parents, Barbara and Edward, for showing me unending support, your faith in me, and your love which I have had since the day I was conceived.

To my prince, Tom, for picking up all the slack without complaint through my illness, and during the course of hour to hour, day by day writing of *Impossible Choices*. For your devotion to our marriage... to me, our daughter, and your secure and abiding love.

To Alice and Big Tom (Grampy) Dooling, for all you do to help care for Kara, your kindness, humor, and unending concern.

To each one of our siblings... brothers, sisters, and in-laws, and nieces and nephews, and all the extended cousins for being there when I needed a friend, for cards, calls and caring about Tom, Kara, and I... for your love. To my one and only sister Mary who gives so much of herself to others.

To my precious little Kara Elizabeth, for putting up with mommy spending long hours sitting at the computer instead of joining you in a game of tickles. For rubbing my shoulders and patting my back at the end of a tiresome day. How I love your tiny kisses that send a sensation throughout my entire body and stay on my cheeks until bedtime. For the incredible joy you put into my life.

To all the aunts and uncles who continue to remember me (us) in prayer, and who have helped us financially: Aunt Kitty, Uncle Howie and Aunt Jackie, Uncle Lawrence, and Aunt Phyllis.

To my loyal friends, Bruce, Julie, and Sheila… Denise, Fran, and Kim, for open arms and ears! For the laughter and spirit you have given me.

To my thoughtful neighbors who are too good to be true… Mary and Bill, Linda and Bob, and Lenny.

To my wonderful team of doctors, nurses, staff, volunteers, and anyone that has taken part in my healthcare… you all are literally keeping me alive!

To all my former employers who are doctors and have given lots of free advice, referrals to all the best hospitals, compassion, and concern for my family and I… Andy, Elliot, Mace, and Jay.

To my breast cancer support group who are literally keeping me sane! For all your support, hugs, and tissues, and for sharing your own stories that have inspired me.

To Diane Reagan, a dedicated English teacher who volunteered to edit and prepare my manuscript for my publisher.

To Noreen Wise, my editor and publisher (now friend) who saw a rainbow and gave of herself… more than her expertise and knowledge, and allowed my dream to come true.

To Mike the mailman… You are the best!

An abundance of thanks to You, God, and my baby angel Jenna Rose, and of course my April Angel.

And to you, my readers. Enjoy! May you be inspired to be true to your dreams and live every day to the fullest! And may all your storms be followed by rainbows.

.

My Diary

December 25, 1970

Dear Diary,

Hello from me. This is my first time writing in a diary. I am nine years old. I got my diary today for Christmas from my sister Mary. We all had so much fun opening gifts and filling our bellies with a big feast! I think I'm going to like my new diary. Mary says that diaries are for secrets. I have a big secret. It's about my mother. I think she is ill or something. She doesn't act right. Dad calls her weird moments "spells." So when Mom is having one of her spells, I try to hide. I don't know what this terrible disease is, but it changes her mood as quickly as a scene in a play. Her behavior is really strange. Sometimes she thinks we are trying to kill her. I don't want to kill Mom. I love Mom. I don't want to know this stranger. She is surely not the warm and caring mother I know. She is not the same person who hugs and kisses me, and calls me her precious angel. This woman is not kind and loving. She is scary. She is angry and hurtful. She is not my mother. I can't do anything right around this person. I can't talk with her. It's like my own mother died. I wish she'd come back to me.

My real mother is a beautiful woman inside and out. She is full of joy and laughter. She is kind and loving in every way. Everyone loves her because she loves everyone. I hear people say my real mother has so much wisdom and faith. I'm not sure what wisdom and faith are, but I know they're good things because my dad says they are. She is gentle and forgiving. Family and friends like to come to our home because they can always enjoy a delicious meal. Mom is a fabulous cook. Our house smells of good food. I am always with my mother. Folks say we are inseparable. As the youngest of six, she takes me every where she goes. I am always at her side. I love being with her. But I don't like being with her when she is having a spell. When I get older, I'm not going to have any spells. I'm going to have a little girl and I won't say scary things to her.

February 10, 1971

My friend Sheila had a sleep over last night. Sheila is already ten years old—one year older than me. Sheila is my best friend. I've known her since first grade. She has long black hair and wears it long and loose, just like me. Only mine is dirty blond. We are both short and we like a lot of the same things: we both want to have kids, and we both love animals. Last night we played house and pretended we were married. Sheila was married to Donny Osmond and I was married to David Cassidy. We made believe that Sheila had three children and I had four. We pretended our kids were in school; we made fake lunches and brushed the girls' hair "just right" for class pictures. I have a poster of David Cassidy in my room and I practiced kissing him on the poster. Sheila practiced her kissing on my Donny Osmond album. I like playing house; I like being married with children.

April 23, 1971

Yippee! I'm ten! Mom always makes me my favorite cake on my birthday. Cherry chip with white frosting. Then she decorates it

Impossible Choices

with colored sprinkles and puts my little angel on the top. Mom bought this angel keepsake when I was born, and today she said that I could have her for my very own. Mom finally took it out of the china cabinet and gave her to me to keep in my bedroom. My angel sat on my Christening cake and my First Holy Communion cake. Whenever that angel appears for special events, Mom always says that she's there to bless me for all the years to come! My angel is a delicate piece with a gold halo. The painted colors on her face and gown are now faded. She carries a tiny brown rabbit and she rests on top of a white cloud with worn out gold words: *April Angel*. She has survived my reckless play and carelessness. Mom explained that when she was pregnant with me, she prayed to the angels to give her another girl. That's why she bought the angel... to pray to. She wanted Mary to have a sister. Mom's always praying to someone in heaven for something. When Mom was pregnant with Mary, the story goes... that because she already had three boys she prayed every night to the Blessed Mother for a girl, and promised to name the baby after her. Yup, you got it... that's how Mary got her name. And me? Well, I'm named after Mom! I have found the perfect spot for my angel. I'm going to keep her on my night stand so she can watch over me while I sleep. In the morning, she'll be the first thing I see. And I do feel like she watches over me. I like to pray to my April Angel when I get scared... like when Dad drinks or when Mom has a spell.

June 24, 1971

Dear Diary, More secrets! Mom really freaked-out this week! She's been crying for days. I wish I knew why; I want to help her to stop feeling sad. One minute she's sobbing and the next she's freaking-out and screaming. I heard Dad call it a nervous break down. All I know is that some impostor has taken over my mom. I don't know what to do. Sometimes I hide upstairs in my closet or I run out of the house quick as a jack rabbit. I just go walking and cry the whole way. Other times I go to the mall which is right across the street from our house. But usually if I'm crying, I don't want people to see me, so I walk to the cemetery two blocks away. That's a good place to cheer up believe it or not. Sounds super weird, but I stroll along reading the headstones and before you know it, I'm thinking about these people and what kind of lives they lived before they died. Plus, the graveyard is so peaceful. Not much fussing and yelling in a graveyard. Hah! The trees are very green in summer and colorful in autumn. I don't go there in the winter if snow is on the ground. But I sure do enjoy it when the trees are budding or the leaves are in flames with fall colors. I choose the biggest tree I can find to sit underneath, and write in my private diary. Yep, it sure is an old familiar place for me to go and dream. When I see a headstone of a young person, I realize how lucky I am. Like I could be buried six feet under and not enjoying this warm sunny day, or be an orphan. Jeez, not having Mom at all would be worse than she is right now.

Mom has to go into the hospital. It is going to be hard to lose her because I love her so much. It will seem like an eternity while she is gone. Our house will be so empty without her. I'll miss her voice. I'll miss her smell. I'll miss the way she brushes my hair. While she's in the hospital, my brother Eugene and I will have to stay in Connecticut with our big brother Russ and his wife Ann. Gene and I are the youngest. I call him Eugene Christopher Columbus Goyette. His middle name is Christopher, because he was born on Columbus Day. He doesn't like me to play with his name like that, so now I just call him Gene even though almost everyone else says

Impossible Choices

Eugene. When I was much younger, I used to call him Nugene because I couldn't say his name right. Well, Nugene Christopher Columbus and I get passed around a bit whenever Mom goes nuts or if Dad is drinking. Once in a while we are sent to our Aunt Betty's house, and other times we just stay home. It is hard to know what will happen next. Sometimes both parents act up at the same time. All I can say is that Mom cries a lot and dad drinks and yells a lot… And me? I walk and write a lot. And I daydream, too… it seems that the worse the day, the bigger my dreams. I imagine all sorts of hopes and fantasies. I have fun doing this! I have learned that if I can stay cheerful on the inside by keeping all my thoughts happy, I can make those terrible feelings go away. I have to remember that I can do this with my hopes and dreams… and the biggest one of all is that one day I will have a perfect family.

August 18, 1971

I'm happy that Sheila is still my friend. She moved to Medford, Massachusetts, but we still spend all our school vacations together. We still play house, only now she is married to Robert Wagner and I am married to Bobby Sherman—movie stars instead of singers. They are both very handsome. I still pretend to have four children. I have two boys and two girls. I have to get a picture of Bobby Sherman the next time I'm at Bradlees so I can practice my kissing. Mom is forever telling me to tie my wild hair back! She says I look like a gypsy. I think gypsies are pretty. Sheila wears hers loose too. We try to look like Mary. It's nice having a big sister to copy especially when mine is so pretty. Mary sits on a chair by the ironing board, lays out her long locks, and puts a paper bag on top. Sheila and I take turns ironing her hair. Then we watch Mary dress and put on her make-up. Mom and Dad only let her wear a little bit of eye shadow and blush. After Mary leaves to go out on a date, Sheila and I are left with the two Bobs—Robert and Bobby.

April 24, 1972
Even though Mom is having a lot of problems, Dad is still getting plastered. That big bottle of Italian red wine sits at the kitchen table with Dad till he passes out. Sometimes he is thirsty for whiskey, and that's when he gets loud and mean. I can't really tell if Dad drinks because of mom's spells or if she freaks-out because of dad's drinking. Maybe they are both crazy. I hear that crazy people do weird things. Mom and Dad do lots of weird things. I'm sure that there is no hope for Dad or for us. If I'm eleven, that means I have seven more years of this. Can I survive two thousand five hundred and fifty-five more days of living nightmares?

My mother sent me to a counselor who said that Dad has alcoholism. So now Dad has alcoholism and Mom has spells of depression. The social worker lady told me that Dad can be treated. She says that even the worst of alcoholics can be helped. I know that she is trying to give me hope, but I don't believe this woman. Dad drinks a real lot and he's already been to many detox centers. It is unbelievable when he goes to the bar and gets drunk on the very same day he gets out of a rehab. I wonder how he can do this to himself and his family. I get so angry with him. I have stopped speaking to him. I make any excuse not to be home. When I am home, I don't eat at the same table with him. I eat many dinners alone up in my room. Geno does the same thing. (Now everyone, even me, calls him Geno.) Mom prepares the nicest meals, and we are selfish enough to ruin them by not eating together. During these times, I hate my own dad. I don't feel it's right to hate your father. I even told Mom this and I begged her to get a divorce. She only tells

Impossible Choices

me not to say such things about my father, that it is the drink that cursed him.

Our nights are filled with suspense. I go to sleep with my headphones on and blast Bob Seger so that I don't hear Dad yelling and screaming. Also *Hold Out* by Jackson Brown and *Anticipation* by Carlie Simon. Music is a great big boost to my state of mind. If I can just hang on for one more day, everything will be okay. One day is just twenty-four hours. If I tell myself this every day, maybe I really will survive seven more years. Once in a while I turn the volume down to listen for a bang. Mary is the real lookout. She sits at the top of the stairs like a watchdog. She can fly down the steps three or four at a time. She tries to stop Dad from breaking up the house. It seems Mary gets the brunt of this chaos because she is the oldest sibling at home right now. Poor Mary plays mother, father, and sister. She must be very tired. I think she is brave. I am thankful she is here to help take care of things. When my brothers Kenny and Paul are home from college break, I feel safe. However, the boys occasionally fight with dad and this upsets Mom so much. I don't know what is worse: being alone, or having the boys home to fight with Dad.

I seem to cry a lot these days. I have a huge outburst then I get hold of myself and do something constructive. I can't get overwhelmed by what's happening here at home. It will consume me if I let it! No way! I'm not going to let that happen to me… I can make it one more day. I have my dear diary to escape to, and speed strolling to the cemetery, or to church when it's empty. I like to go there and just sit in the pew. The doors are not usually locked until evening. It's heavenly inside! Hee hee. I mean real quiet. I like quiet.

Barbara Dooling

June 6, 1972

Wow, last night was a real doozy. Dad was very drunk and Paul had a big fight with him. They were really screaming. Nights like this, I lay awake for a long time. I cry into my pillow. It was hard getting up for school this morning. I never speak to anyone about these frightful evenings and I suspect neither does the rest of my family. We don't discuss things at home either. I have a lot of friends, and I love going to their houses after school. It is especially nice to be invited to stay for dinner. I can laugh and forget about my father. Sometimes my friends and I go for pizza at Papa Gino's. That's loads of fun because we can put quarters in the juke box and select our favorite songs. I always pick: *I Think I Love You* by David Cassidy, *Johnny Angel* by Shelley Fabares or *Sugar Sugar* by The Archies. Mom doesn't like me staying out so much. I am sure she feels like her family is falling apart. As much as I like being away from home, I never stop worrying about Mom. Even Dad. I always wonder what kind of mess I will walk into when I get home. Many things get broken, but we clean everything up, one mess at a time. Part of the clean up is searching through Dad's pockets when he passes out. We figure if he has no money, he can't buy more booze. We also hide his bottles or dump them out down the sink. It never stops him though. I'm glad that Dad doesn't hit Mom or hit us. He just breaks things in the house.

My Journal

April 22, 1973

    I just got this new journal for my twelfth birthday. Even though I received a lot of nice gifts, this one is my favorite. Mary gave it to me because she knows how much I love my Diary. I'm going to write all about my life in this journal. I was born on April 22, 1961, the same year that our family moved into our house on Washington Street in Dedham. Our house is a good size for a family of eight. We have two bathrooms. This is a big deal when you have four brothers and one sister. It's a bit easier to get the bathroom nowadays since Russ and Kenny have moved out. They are the oldest, and I really miss them. I love them a whole bunch! They are very different from each other. Russ has real short hair. He and Ann have a sweet baby girl named Kimberly after Kimberly Ave in Connecticut where they live. It's hard to believe that I'm already an auntie. I always thought aunts were old people.

    Kenny has really, really long hair and a wild looking beard and mustache. Dad says Russ is "collegiate" whatever that means. I don't know why he calls Russ this and Kenny a "hippy" because they both go to college. I think it has something to do with the kind of clothes they each wear. Russ always wears white shirts and ties. Kenny wears bell bottom jeans that have patches all over them. All I know is that Dad got real mad at Kenny when he patched the seat of his

Barbara Dooling

dungarees with the American flag. Dad said he shouldn't sit on the flag like that. And Kenny likes to wear Dad's old army jacket—the long wool coat that is one ugly color green. But it does have fancy gold buttons and some kind of colorful stripes sewed on the shoulders. I think those bands mean something special. Dad says Kenny should fight in a war and understand what the flag and that army coat are all about. So Kenny still wears the coat, only Mom changed all those shiny buttons to black ones, and she took the sharpest scissors she has and ripped those stripes off so Kenny could wear the coat and still keep peace with Dad. Frankly, I think that Kenny is the peace keeper. Kenny taught me how to make a peace sign with my fingers. He always says, "Peace, Man. Peace and Love, Brother." He even smoked something called a "peace pipe." I thought only the Indians did that. But for some reason Kenny says he doesn't smoke the peace pipe anymore. He doesn't like any kind of war. I don't know why Dad gets so grumpy about all this stuff. I was so scared that Russ or Kenny would have to fight in that Vietnam War because I didn't want them to get "kilt." If they did, I don't know how I would live without them.

Kenny says that he was a flower child back in the 1960's, and he went to a place called Woodstock. This was where a ton of people and hippies had a great big party with music. Both Russ and Kenny are good at playing the guitar, but they don't sing the same kinds of songs. Russ plays something called folk music like songs by Peter, Paul, and Mary and Kenny plays *Rocky Raccoon* by the Beatles. I like listening to both of them strum any kind of music. It's kind of funny how Russ and Kenny are not at all alike, but I love them both the exact same. The only time I get mad at Russ is when he punishes me when I say a swear word. Like the time I said S—T. He made me stand and hold my arms out straight, then he placed a

Impossible Choices

huge dictionary across my arms, and I had to hold it for a really long time. If I drop it, then he just gets a bar of soap and washes out my mouth. So I don't say bad words a whole lot—at least not in front of Russ. Once when Geno said a naughty word, he had to hold the Bible which is just as fat and heavy.

Even though there are four bedrooms in our house I don't have my own room. I don't mind sharing a room with Mary because she is the greatest sister anyone could ever have. When I want to be alone, I sit inside our nice bright sun porch. Our yard is very big with lots of fruit trees. We have a huge grape vine that grows the biggest purple grapes you ever saw. While all the neighborhood kids are playing tag, we are picking pears, cherries, apples, and grapes. Whenever dad isn't looking, Geno and I have grape fights and smash grapes on each other's heads. The bees buzz around us and I swat at them and scream like some crazy person. Mom puts up pear preserves and makes homemade grape juice and jelly. There are always fruit flies in the kitchen. Mom says they are clean flies. Our house smells delicious and all the neighbors stop by for a jar of Mom's preserves. I don't know where she finds the time to do it. We always have fresh fruits and vegetables to eat.

Mom says the harvest is the best time of year. I like it too, because after the harvest, the holidays are quick to follow. Oh, how I love the holidays! Mom is Italian. She cooks the most wonderful dinners. Mom starts with something called antipasto. The grown-ups love antipasto. It's a dish filled with lots of weird things. Mom makes homemade manicotti, eggplant parmesan, and veal cutlets. After all that, then come the turkey, stuffing, and vegetables. The food just keeps appearing in front of our eyes. What a howl! For desert, there are always homemade pies, never store bought. There is Easter bread if it's Easter. At Christmas, there are pizzella cookies,

Barbara Dooling

and biscotti, all made from scratch. Mom bakes for weeks for each holiday. It is fun to help flip the pizzella iron over the stove flames. This year Mom finally got an electric pizzella iron. The house is warm and sweet smelling for days. I always help Mom with the decorating. We make a lot of our own Christmas ornaments and decorations. Besides the ones we make, we have some very old-fashioned ornaments. I want a home just like this. I want to be a mother, and have a little girl like me to help with everything. I wonder if I will fall in love someday.

May 3, 1974

Wow. Jeez. Ahmmm... How do I write this without blushing? Another secret! Today was the hugest day of my entire life (or so I'm told by Mary). It's the day of my first P—D! WHOOOA. I'm not sure I like this. In fact I'm sure I don't. Well, I'm like... excited and all, but this is not real fun to deal with. Hmmm. Yep, I guess I'm psyched that I finally got it. I called Mary right away. She has her own apartment now and I just love visiting. I'm glad she was home. She was happy to hear my news. She's thrilled. She wants me to tell Mom right away. Ugh! I hope Mom doesn't tell Dad. Ugh! I just don't want too many people to know, especially my brothers and Dad. Yet at the same time, I can't wait to tell Sheila and my other girlfriends. But God, I wouldn't want the boys in school to know. This is kind of embarrassing, and I'm just a bit scared. You mean this comes every month? Can I still go swimming? Last summer, Sheila's mother told her that she couldn't go in the water when she has her period. Well, Mary says that's just not so. Oh this is like... wicked intense. I think getting boobs is more important and a bigger deal than getting a period!

Impossible Choices

September 24, 1974

Okay so, my face is breaking out since I've started my period. Mom tells me that I am a woman now. I don't feel like a woman. Jeez, I'm only thirteen. I feel more like a brand new teenager who doesn't like what's happening to her body. These blemishes are unsightly and these cramps from my so called "friend" are not very friendly at all. Will any of the boys I know want to take me to the junior high school dance? I wonder. Mom says I'm her Miss America, and Dad calls me his princess. Sometimes they both call me their Barbie doll. I don't see any zits on Miss America, Cinderella, or Barbie. And where did these long lanky arms and legs come from? I feel so clumsy. Will I ever get bosoms like Barbie? I just don't like my body right now. I feel like a monkey with all this hair on my legs. So I tried to use Dad's razor, but cut myself real bad. Mom gave me her electric razor. Seems to me I'm going to need a lawnmower. Mary said I should be using deodorant underneath my armpits now. I broke the news to her that Mom's been having me use antiperspirant since… you know… three months ago. I have to shave the pits now too cause the hair gets long enough to braid. Not to worry Mary, Mom says the underarm spray is as important as a daily vitamin. She makes sure I don't skip. It's weird, I was like wondering where that odor was coming from. I was so grossed out that it was actually "ME"! Nope, I never miss the "morning squirt before I put on the shirt."

I just know when people talk to me they are staring at my pimples. What's with this nose of mine? Mom said that when I was a baby I had the most tiny button nose. Now the family resemblance is with Pinocchio! I feel so gawky. I'm just not pretty at all. Why am I ugly? Will I change like the duckling? Hope so. I really hope I get to that dance. Maybe I'll meet some new friends.

Barbara Dooling

I have a crush on a very cute guy in my English class—Matthew. He has olive skin and dark brown, wavy hair and he's short like me. Matt sits in front of me in the third row. He's always talking to me, but I don't think he really likes me… you know, in that way. He hasn't caught on that I wish he'd ask me to the school dance. Boys are so dumb. It takes a sledgehammer to wake them up. I'll just have to pray to my April Angel to open his eyes.

Dedham Junior High School is huge compared to my old grammar school. There seem to be thousands of kids that I don't know. But there are lots of boys and I like that. Alex is in my homeroom and he's always flirting with me at our lockers. It's fun to get all this attention. I wonder how old Mom and Dad were when they got married. Hmmm, maybe I'll marry Matthew. He's so sweet. Mom says I shouldn't be in such a rush with my life. There's too much to look forward to: high school, college, and careers. Mom wants me to go to college because she never did. She wishes a lot of things for me that she never had. I guess that's what moms do. Me, I just want to have a family of my own. I love my brothers and my sister. We have a lot of fun together. Geno and I listen to albums together. We like the same music. Mary teaches me how to match my clothes, and how to put on make-up. Paul and Kenny are my older brothers. They give me rides in Dad's car and take me all over Dedham. Kenny plays the guitar and sings to me. My brothers and my sister are wicked cool. They take good care of me. Mary lets me tag along with her when she hangs out down at "the pit." The pit is this big park that has hills and trees all around it. It's like a dug out park so everyone calls it the pit. Seems like all the kids in Dedham hang out there. The boys—that's what I always call my brothers—are very protective. I think it's great to be a member of a big family. Someday… after I meet the perfect guy, I will have a great awesome

Impossible Choices

big family too. The man I marry will be very special! Meeting the perfect guy… that's "happily ever after" for me.

February 6, 1975

Tonight I was at my friend Suzanne's house, listening to music and hanging out with her two brothers John and David. I like her parents. For one thing, they are a lot younger than mine. They even seem to like our music. Suzanne wears her mother's clothes. Mrs. H and Sue act like they are best friends. Maybe because they are. I sure love my mom, but it's hard to be friends with the stranger she becomes when her mood changes. One day I am going to have a daughter who will be my best friend. John and David are younger than us, but they're pretty neat guys. We made brownies, then pigged out on them, and played cards. Their parents weren't home, so we could really blast the tunes. Suey, David, and I actually got up and danced to practically every song on *Bat Out of Hell* by Meat Loaf. It was way cool. For a few awesome hours I was able to forget my anguish over my family. I just let it all go and set my spirit free! Then Sue's mom came back and said it was time to wrap up our little party; she drove me home. When we pulled up to my house, there was an ambulance parked in our driveway. It was snowing and it looked as though Dad had been shoveling. I jumped out of the car and told Mrs. H that it was okay for her to leave. She waved bye with a funny expression on her face.

Dad was inside the ambulance getting checked out. I cried, "Dad, are you okay? Daddy, oh Daddy, please be okay!" I thought maybe he had fallen on the ice. Worse than that, I was terrified that my dad had had a heart attack. I thought it was odd that the ambulance was not taking dad to the hospital. Then Dad sort of stumbled out by himself. And he was staggering toward the house.

Barbara Dooling

He said, "I'm okay, honey." When I hugged him I could smell stale alcohol. Although it was dark, I could see the drunken look in his eyes from the streetlight. As he spoke, I saw his twisted mouth and heard the slurring of his speech. Dad was smashed. My heart was still racing from the scare. I was shaking from the cold and the fear of losing him because I really do love my father. I was so angry and yet so relieved. I screamed at Dad, but it was no use. Whenever I tell him how horrible he is when he drinks, his guilt only makes him drink more.

Mom called Aunt Betty while Dad sat slumped over at the kitchen table. Aunt Betty came right away and they took Dad to rehab again to "dry out." I feel ashamed because I never miss Dad when he's in some hospital. I don't want him to come home at all because it is so peaceful without him. I wish I didn't feel this way, but it's the truth. Things are just so mixed up in my mind. What if Dad had had a heart attack tonight? What if he had died?! I realize that I really do love Dad and I will miss him. It's the disease that I hate. We all love Dad and we love each other very much. It is this love that carries us through these dreadful days. Oh, I pray to my little April Angel that this time Dad stays sober. Tonight I'm going to sleep with her underneath my pillow. She'll be safe and close to me there.

March 15, 1975

So far so good. Dad's been able to stay away from the bottle. I'm so grateful! It seems like a miracle. I had to tell Suzanne a little bit about that night when the ambulance was in front of my house. She and her mother were curious. Don't know how I've managed to put that awful experience out of my mind. Sue thinks I have nerves of steel. She said that even at school I handle things differently than

Impossible Choices

other kids. Like when that creep Lank Smith was teasing Marge Wheeler. I sat with Marge in the cafeteria, day after day, and ate lunch with her because no one else would. I told that buffoon that he wasn't a threat to me. What a jerk. Marge thanked me for standing by her. I just explained that what doesn't destroy you will make you stronger (that's a famous saying by a famous psychiatrist). Sue and Marge acted sort of surprised that this was my reaction. I must confess it seems so minor compared to things going on in my house. But like I said, Dad's been great so I've just been enjoying these quiet days. It's like getting to know who Dad really is. He gave me one of his old weightlifting trophies to keep. Now that's strong! Dad was into weight lifting when he was younger! He showed me some of his other trophies and lots of silver and gold medals. Wow, how cool is that?!

April 28, 1975

Our peace and quiet was short lived! As if puberty and adolescence aren't hard enough, Dad's gone back to hitting the bottle. Seems like more than ever. He is so unpredictable. I seem to be crying all the time. I'm in the eighth grade and it's such a confusing time in my life. My emotions have been more extreme than ever before. At the smallest incident or upset, I run to my room, slam the door and burst into tears. And it seems that while Dad is struggling with his addiction, Mom is fighting her own battle with "Depression." I've now learned that's what it's called. I can understand it I guess. Who wouldn't be depressed… like I can even see me getting down. But whenever we have a bad day, I run to my room and try with all my might to think about the good days. I'm trying this cool scientific experiment to see if I think hard enough about happy days, keep those vivid memories in the front of my

Barbara Dooling

mind, that I can actually make them come back to me. I'll make a go of it and see how the ball bounces. Never mind the ball, I'm determined to throw those ideas around in my head like a boomerang. Every day I'll do this until I have a happy family. It's way cool! I am learning that when I think of these wonderful thoughts and hopes, that my mind can't be troubled by sad stuff at the same time. I can take myself far away to a place over the rainbow, and I can wish on all those first stars, the falling stars, and the whole darn galaxy. I feel better already. I always wish the same thing—to get Mom and Dad well. Why can't our family be happy like Sue's or Rosie's? Why can't we sit around the table laughing and telling jokes? One day we will. That's my hope. One day I will have that.

June 10, 1975

This day is filled with warm sunshine in a cloudless blue sky. I'm sitting on the lush grounds at Endicott Estate—one of my favorite places in the whole wide world. It's kind of a long walk from my house, but worth it. People come here to have picnics, play football, and just hang around. I visit to write, to think, and to dream. The town bought this grand mansion and all this grass! Once in a while, on a Saturday or a Sunday, you can catch a wedding! Wouldn't I love to get married at such a beautiful spot. I have plopped myself on top of a small hill where I can capture a wonderful view. I can't even imagine only one family living in that huge manor. I can just picture it in the olden days—pulling up in a horse drawn carriage to attend a ball! Maybe someday I will, only it will be my wedding.

January 3, 1976

WOW! My friend Karen at school was crying hysterically, just like Mom usually does during one of her melt downs. She was upset

Impossible Choices

because she thought her dad was mad at her because she didn't have a perfect race during an indoor track meet. She lost it because her father didn't think she was trying hard enough. Hmmm... I was standing right there and her father didn't sound that upset to me. He just said that it seemed like she wasn't trying her best. He asked her if everything was all right. How nice of him to even notice—to even ask. At least her dad goes to the meets. Mine has to work, and I'm not so sure I'd even want him there anyway.

Karen explained to her dad that she had tried her hardest, but that she was having a bad day! (Her locker was broken into, and her boyfriend's best friend had teased her by making a mess of her books and papers and throwing them all over the hall. At lunch, she spilled coke on her silk blouse. Then she forgot her best track sneakers, and had to call her mother to bring them to school in time for the bus that took us to the meet. She had a fight with her boyfriend about something—who knows what, probably his friend. And to top it off, she placed second in that race, which is why I guess her father made the comment.) I think placing in a race at all is awesome! HMMMM...

I must be growing up in more ways than just getting my period. This would have been "THE BEST DAY OF MY LIFE." I'm used to picking up after someone who smashes furniture, my clothes are hand-me-downs from Mary so they're already stained, and I can't forget my favorite sneakers 'cause I only have one pair, and I wear them to school every day! But if I did leave them at home, we don't have a car and Mom doesn't drive anyway, so she couldn't get them to me. Dad takes the subway to work, and he gets home too late to ever make it to any of my track meets, and forget practices. Oh yah, and I don't have a boyfriend to fight with. See? My millions of hours are spent daydreaming and praying for days just like Karen's. Trade

Barbara Dooling

ya, Karen! Wanna switch places for a day?

April 24, 1976

My three older brothers no longer live at home. Russ is married, and Kenny and Paul are still away in college. Mary is still at her apartment. Geno and I are still at home and we're now in high school. I'm fifteen—a freshman. I'm getting much better at staying cool. Maintain an even strain, right? Gotta stay cool! I see how some kids at school act. They are wicked partiers getting drunk or drugged out! I wonder if they have a bad situation at home, too. I think they are just like Dad... hooked on something. I have absorbed myself in my studies and after-school sports. I've become quite a "jockette" on the track team. All that exhilarating hiking in the graveyard has really paid off.

Our team won the "Bay State championship" this year, with me placing first and second at many of those track meets. My racing times were good enough to be eligible for state competitions where I won a silver and a bronze medal. I have excelled academically and in track. Mentally it has been a great way to relieve the stress from home. I have become a woman and I realize that it is time for me to learn ways of coping with my family problems. Now I'm trying to open up to friends and relatives about the truth. I'm not going to hide or be ashamed of my parents anymore. I have begun talking with Mom and Dad about their illnesses. I've confronted them firmly, and told them that I would not stand by and watch them destroy themselves, each other, and their family. There is far too much love to let that happen. I know that I can't make my parents recover because this is something they must work out themselves. But I can begin to change myself. I am learning how to help myself deal with their problems. I'm so thankful for my

Impossible Choices

journal. Writing things down makes me feel better; I can validate my feelings. I have learned to talk about my parents' illnesses with them and my siblings. Once we are all talking rationally, perhaps it will be easier to come up with strategies to help Mom and Dad.

I keep going to our church and praying to God to make my mother and father better. I pray to have faith and hope that we will someday have peace in our home. And I pray to rid myself of the guilt that I feel because at times, I do not like the people my parents have become. If they were not so wonderful and special I would not miss them as much when they change. Dad always says to pick ourselves up after a fall. He says that when the trellis falls, the roses still try to climb. I wish Dad would listen to his own advice.

April 10, 1977

It's Easter Sunday and a beautiful spring day! I'm in the back yard with the sun and the budding trees. Two more months and school will be out for summer! I'm thinking about my birthday—only twelve more days. I can't wait to be sixteen! Wow! Sixteen seems a million years older than thirteen. I can learn to drive! Mom and Dad will let me date boys! My new weekend curfew will be ten o'clock! Next year I'll be a junior! High school is the best! I love all my classes. I still have zits, but I have learned how to camouflage them with make-up. I finally have breasts. It took them long enough to grow. Awe Jeez, is this it? Will they get any bigger? I am still on the track team and it's so cool. I love being a part of the whole team. I've made so many new friends. We sing and get rowdy on the bus while we drive to our track meets. This gets us hyped up for the meets. We sing *Doing it Our Way*, that song that they sing on the Laverne and Shirley Show. I just love that song. We are like a family.

Barbara Dooling

Like the Cunninghams on *Happy Days* or *The Brady Bunch*! Yep, one big happy bunch... no yelling and drinking and spells. I love school because it's like a never ending social event. I mostly hang with Elizabeth, Patricia, Joan, and Suzanne. The boys at Dedham High are very shy. (Being in sports, I've met a lot of boys.) I'm not allowed out on school nights except when I have track meets. Mom and Dad are sending me to Colonial Williamsburg in Virginia for my sixteenth birthday. I can't believe they're letting me go. It will be my first time flying on a plane and being away from home. I'm going with Elizabeth and Patricia. We're going to stay with Patricia's sister who lives in Virginia. I can't wait!

April 16, 1977

Okay... I'm in Williamsburg! Survived the first flight. All three of us had never been on an airplane; we were a mess. But we are safe and sound now, and actually the trip was very exciting, especially the feeling from the extreme velocity. During takeoff, I felt like a paper clip being slung from a rubber band! *Petoo Petoo Petoo!*

I've never seen so many flowering trees. I can recognize Dogwoods and Magnolia because Dad always points these out back home and around Boston. The Dogwood trees look just as though they are kissing the sky, and the magnificent Magnolia have large pink and white tulip-like cups. There are also many cherry blossoms, and other trees that I can't even name... all bursting with delicate blooming flowers. And I've seen a ton of lemon-colored daffodils! Everything is so bright and cheerful. Our itinerary for the next few days will be: Busch Gardens, Colonial Williamsburg, Jamestown, Virginia Beach, and The College of William and Mary! YAY! I can't wait. Elizabeth and Patricia have insisted on celebrating my birthday with a small cake since the real event is just days away.

Impossible Choices

Spent our first evening here blowing out my seventeen candles (one for good luck) and laughing about the bumpy but safe landing.

April 22, 1977

Yahoo, sixteen! Friday night back at home! What a wild and fabulous party my friends threw for me. Awesome! Everyone gathered at my house while Elizabeth and Patricia took me shopping for new track sneakers. That was their gift to me. So while we were at the Walpole Mall, Suzanne, Joan and Rosie decorated with streamers and balloons. Sheila and a whole gang of kids came down from Medford to crash my bash! There was Julie and Bruce, John, Michael, Mark, Chris, Derb, and Zap. I have no idea what the last two kids' real names are—that's what everyone calls them. The Medford kids call me Dedhamite. I've been getting to know them on weekends when I venture out to see Sheila. I take a bus from Dedham to Forest Hills in West Roxbury, then the orange line all the way from the Hills to Medford. Bruce has a car so he's the one who picks me up at the station. Mom goes absolutely berserk because she worries about my safety on the subway.

They hang around at a corner called The Pipe, and for my birthday they gave me a T-shirt that says "Honorary Pipe Member" on the front, and "Dedhamite" on the back. I'm honored all right! This was the best party. I think Mom and Dad are great for letting my friends have the house. We played loud music and danced to: The Rolling Stones, The Eagles, The Who, Pink Floyd, Aerosmith, Bad Company, and The Beatles. God, it's past midnight and everyone just left! We had such a blast! It was just so exciting… and on their way out, all the guys kissed me and wished me the happiest birthday! They were all just friendly smooches, but still…

Barbara Dooling

August 23, 1977

Summer break! Here I sit among the flat rocks of the jetty. The ocean is noisy with crashing waves and loud hungry seagulls hovering above. I've something to share. Some really big news! And I'm going to put it right here in my journal. Sweet sixteen, but I've been kissed!

Mom and Dad always rent a cottage for a couple of weeks during summer vacation. Since Mom's family spent their summers in Plymouth on White Horse Beach, that's where she likes to take us. I always get to bring a friend, and I always bring Sheila. She's still my best friend since first grade, even after moving to Medford. Geno, Sheila, and I walk the beach together every day. We have a nice sea-glass collection and lots of pretty shells and rocks.

That's how we met Craig. He was skimming stones across the water. Craig is a year younger than me and he's cute. We all went miniature golfing together and Craig asked me out! I've never been out with anyone before. I was ecstatic; Sheila coached me on what to say. She's never gone out with anyone either, but somehow she had lots of perfect suggestions. Now I need more HELP! HELP! HELP! Craig is so nice and Geno likes him, too.

It happened right there on the beach, Craig kissed me—on the lips. We were sitting on the beach watching the waves, and Craig just leaned over and kissed me! He scooched real close, and we held hands after that dreamy kiss. I think I'm in love already. I feel like Lezal in the movie, *The Sound of Music*. She was in love at sixteen, too, and she danced the night away in a gazebo with her charming boyfriend. This is going to be the shortest romance in history. I have to go back home in ten days and I'll probably never see Craig again. We exchanged addresses, but he lives in Connecticut. Since his parents just rented a cottage, he's not sure when or if he'll

Impossible Choices

get back to Plymouth. I don't know whether I should be feeling ecstatic or bawling my eyes out.

April 23, 1978

Another birthday... Mary gave me another journal for this school trip to Bermuda! The Junior Class Trip. April vacation, and I'm here with Elizabeth, Rosie, and Joan. Bermuda is another world! It's beautiful. I'm sipping my first Pina Colada on a pink sand beach. The turquoise ocean is warm and relaxing. You can see tropical fish and colorful corral right through to the bottom. At home the ocean is very dark and cold. Last night we went to a nightclub for the first time. The music was so loud that it made my heart pound. We were all asked to dance many times. I did my very best. The night went on forever. When we got back to The Elbow Beach Hotel, we strolled along the soft, sandy beach in the warm night air. It will be hard to leave this dream place and go home. Dad always says there is so much to experience in the world. He says to see our own country first. Now I understand what he means about it being such a great opportunity! I can't wait. I never realized the world has this much to offer. I'm going to grab every bit of it that I can. Until now, I've just been a little dot in a little dot town in a little dot state. Times, they are changing... I can feel it in the air tonight...

May 26, 1978

Sitting here on my bed, looking at my prom gown still hanging on my closet door. It needs to be dry-cleaned. My nosegay rests in a bowl of water on my bureau. It is still fresh after a week. Double-dated with Geno for the junior prom. He took Suzanne. I went with Scott. Scott's a really nice guy in my chemistry class. We aren't going out or anything, but we are always chatting about failing this class!

Barbara Dooling

We help each other with homework problems. It was so nice of Scott to ask me to the prom! I said yes, but I made sure he understood that we aren't dating. I don't want to lead him on or anything. We're just friends.

Geno drove Dad's big brown station wagon. What a great night. The prom was held at the Hyatt Regency in Cambridge which is pretty fancy! Scott and I had a blast, but slow dancing was weird. As I looked around at other couples, they were snugly wrapped together. Plenty of guys clinging to girls' waists; girls with their heads nestled gently against the guy's shoulder. Some were kissing. I guess it was just awkward for me, kind of like slow dancing with my own brother. I sure hope Scott didn't feel too funny. Geno really made my night with his jokes and sharp dancing. I kept an eye on him and followed all his moves. Everyone looked so nice, even me! I sat out in the sun all weekend so I would have a tan. I basted with baby oil and cooked myself! Dad yelled that I was going to get skin cancer. He's always yelling… even if he's not drinking…

The day after the prom, I went to White Horse Beach in Plymouth with Elizabeth, Patricia, Joan, and Suzanne. We staked some prime beach space and did what girls do best: laughed and talked; talked and laughed. The weather turned cold and windy, but we didn't seem to mind. There was practically no one else on the beach. We talked about our prom night and boys. We shared secrets about who we wanted to date. The ocean was so lovely. It's such a great spot to get together. It's a super place to come and think when I need to think. Somewhere to dance or run. A place to laugh or cry. This will be my special refuge all right. I really love it. The perfect spot to dream. I'm not dreaming much about a big career. I don't know why, but I don't think about going to college. I know my parents will be so disappointed. Although I do pretty well in my

Impossible Choices

studies at school, I don't feel that I want to go. I don't know if I'm being lazy about it. Dad's drinking doesn't make it easy to study. But I can't use that for an excuse. If I really want to, I could do it. Seems like all I think about is getting married and having a family. I want to live in the country in a big old Victorian house with a white picket fence. I want my kids to have a dog and a cat… maybe a rabbit, too. Wow, I don't even have a boyfriend, never mind a husband to be in this picture. Ah well, some FINE day.

April 29, 1979

You are not going to believe what Julie, Bruce, Mark and I did. Hang on to your chair for this one: We drove all the way to Florida by ourselves for spring break. Whoa! For real. It was Mr. Toad's wild ride for sure! Geno and Paul helped me scrape together the cash. I'm amazed that Mom and Dad let me go. Four crazy friends driving to Orlando for a vacation at Disney World. I've never laughed so much in my life. We were goofing around the whole trip. Bruce and Mark are a real comical team like Laurel and Hardy. They also remind me of the two characters from *The Odd Couple*. Bruce is like Felix Unger and Mark is Oscar Madison. Put them together in a small hotel room, and Broadway better get ready for some stiff competition. Hysterical! Since the four of us shared a room, Julie and I slept in one bed and the guys had to share the other one! Bruce drew an imaginary line separating the sides. All night long you could hear him yelling at Mark, "You're touching me… you're over the line… No touching… Get on your own side." Bruce sleeps like a corpse with his hands neatly folded across his chest and Mark is all over the bed. Every time Mark turned, he would spring his whole body up and pounce back down onto the mattress taking the blanket and sheet with him. Of course Bruce went out of his mind! So Julie and I were entertained day and night. We also entertained ourselves by dining and dancing, swimming in the warm ocean waves, and walking miles around the fantasy streets of Disney. I could go on a trip every year if my finances were more accommodating. There is a big adventure on the horizon! Graduation awaits me this May—just a few more weeks away. I'm eighteen years young! I've journeyed through twelve years of school and eighteen years of home-sweet-home! I am ready for life! Bring it on!! I want to travel and see this country.

July 7, 1979

Here I am at White Horse Beach on this hot Saturday. I met a gorgeous guy during The Fourth of July festivities on the beach yesterday. He's twenty. What a body! He has straight feathered hair that sits just over his ears, dirty blond—and a great tan. I'm in love! For real this time. His name is Steve. I hope I see him today. Luck is on my side this time. It's not like when I met Craig. Steve's parents own a cottage on White Horse Beach; he also lives near Dedham. I should be able to bump into him again... hopefully often. This is going to be a New England HOT vacation and I don't mean sunny.

July 14, 1979

Back down to White horse for this weekend. Some of the Medford kids—Sheila and myself included—got a couple of rooms at a motel. We also brought our sleeping bags and camped out right on the beach under the sparkling stars. Steve's here, too. I wasn't sure if I'd see him because when we met, we never exchanged phone numbers. Two long weeks have passed, and I did nothing but think about him. Last night we shared a blanket while sitting around a bonfire! He didn't even go home to his parent's cottage!

Impossible Choices

He stayed with us all night! I had a lot of chaperones so nothing happened! For one thing, Geno came down with us. I don't think Steve would even kiss me, let alone try anything else. Plus there were at least twenty kids camping out with us. Last but not least... I had the family pet with me! Man's best friend, a Belgian Shepherd with a shiny ebony coat, a brown face, and a thick white chest! Yep, that's Neko! He's really Mary's dog, only she can't keep him at her apartment so Mom and Dad have adopted him. Neko stayed by my side all evening. Once everyone settled down to sleep, Neko became my pillow. I was able to rest my head on his warm tummy all night. But not Steve! It was such a riot. Whenever Steve tried to snuggle next to me and steal a part of Neko, that dog growled fiercely. Poor Steve, between Geno and Neko he couldn't kiss me. But most of all, poor me!

July 15, 1979

Today was spent splashing in the frigid ocean waves and playing Frisbee with Steve and Neko! The two are growing on each other. They're both great catchers. Tee hee, hee. Neko is such a beautiful dog. Steve is such a gorgeous guy!

August 4, 1979

Steve took me back to White Horse to spend the day with his mom Elli. She lives at their cottage all summer. I simply adore her! She's very kind and loves to talk. We sat on the beach all day, gabbing about everything and anything! I finally joined Steve in a sand volley ball game! If you remember, I'm not a bad athlete, so I was all over the beach, pounding the ball! Steve was impressed! When it was time to head back to Boston, I thanked his mom for a splendid day! I feel very close to Elli. I think she likes me, too!

Barbara Dooling

August 25, 1979

Wow! Spending lots of leisure time with Steve. Of course our favorite place to play is Plymouth. Steve and I love to walk the entire length of the beach from the bubbling brook to the point. The stream is a rather large rapid of fresh water which comes from a pond and rushes over huge boulders into the salty sea. It is just heavenly; its like bath water compared to the numbing ocean. We choose a flat rock and try to steady ourselves as the swift water rushes over us. I don't mind losing my balance and bumping bodies with Steve. Then it's back to holding hands and hunting for sea glass and unbroken shells! Midday the sand is so hot it's impossible to stand it and we move to the water's edge. This always tempts Steve to push me into the icy, cold waves. When we finally reach the other end of the beach, there are no people at the point. That's where lovers go to kiss! Not even Geno and Neko could save me! But I didn't really want to be rescued! He's such a good kisser! I like the way he holds my head in his hands and gently presses his lips on mine. He even kissed me in my ear! I was tingling all over!

September 15, 1979

I'm vegging out on my bed with the stereo blasting Bob Seger and The Silver Bullet Band. I'm the only one home on this Saturday afternoon. Mom and Dad are out visiting. I've taken down my old posters of David Cassidy and Bobby Sherman, and replaced them with Bob Seger, Led Zepplin, and The Who. I don't try to kiss Bob Seger. God, I can't believe I used to do that! My bedroom is a pigsty. I know I should put away some of these clothes, but I have this sudden urge to write in my journal. Steve and I have been dating all summer. He's two years older than me. How perfect. He is such a

Impossible Choices

nice guy. Everyone likes him, especially me. We have the best conversations. When we go out on a date, we sit for hours in his car just talking and getting to know each other. We discuss our families, music, and the future. He includes me in his future! He hasn't tried anything yet, if you know what I mean. I really like that. Even when we were kissing down the beach, he was a perfect gentleman. Well, maybe not perfect. But really, we've only kissed. Steve says he feels comfortable around me. I honestly believe he's never experienced a relationship like ours. That is, getting to know each other completely before committing ourselves physically. You know.

He had a steady girlfriend last year, before we met. From what he tells me, they dated for a couple of years, and they were sleeping together. I think they were close, but I know that he and I are even closer. Steve says that he feels differently about me than he has felt with any other girl. He explained that he's been able to share his deepest thoughts and secrets with me because I'm easy to talk with. Perhaps we have found something different and special because we haven't slept together yet. I believe Steve feels no pressure to just "do it" for the sake of doing it or for his own satisfaction. I told him it will happen when we are both ready. Seems guys are always ready for you know what. I'm sure Steve is too, but I'm not. I have to wait until I'm totally sure. Absolutely positively ready! I mean, I want to go all the way with him, too, but I want my first time to be incredibly special. I want to be in love, and to make sure he's in love with me. My friends tell me they've heard some guys just tell girls that just to get them into bed. I believe you need time to figure out and make sure if a guy is true to his word. That bothers some guys, but I never cared. I am who I am, and Steve seems to like that. It seems that he was taught the same values.

Barbara Dooling

October 10, 1979

Mom's in one of her crazy, paranoid relapses. Dad's drunk. I can't stand it! One at a time is bad enough, but both on the same day... give me a break! I've had it! They're losing it! I'm losing it! Get me the hell out of here! They are downstairs screaming back and forth with hateful words and foul language. I've got my headphones blasting WBCN radio station and I can still hear them. I have to get to a phone and call Steve to come and pick me up so I can escape. I'll run over to the mall and use the pay phone, then I can wait for Steve at Friendly's. May as well cry my heart out over a hot fudge sundae. Steve is so great and comes to my rescue... a lot!

November 22, 1979

I'm so excited, I just have to write this all here in my journal! Steve actually met the folks today. I've waited four months to introduce them because I would be mortified if a family episode were to break out in front of Steve. I wasn't afraid of what Steve would do because he already knows the worst... he just hasn't seen it LIVE. Steve keeps telling me to get over it. He has wanted to meet my parents for almost 5 months—today was the day. He spent his Thanksgiving dinner with my whole family! Thank God Dad and Mom are doing well... no drinking, screaming, or crying. Whew! It went soooo well! Geno and Steve already know each other, and were talking up a storm. Mary thinks he's gorgeous. Mom said he's cute, too. Dad chewed his ear off, but that's okay... Steve didn't seem to mind. It's official now that Steve has met my parents... feels like we are really a couple!

December 28, 1979

Another spectacular holiday! Two for two... Mom and Dad are

Impossible Choices

holding their own, and Christmas was just the best! Believe it or not, Steve had dinner with my family again. Would you believe Steve's mom Elli and his little brother Cliff joined us? His dad is a fireman and had to work on Christmas Day, so Mom asked Steve to bring them along. What an event!

Our real tree was extra big this year. Mom and I shared the decorating like always. After Mom's scrumptious Italian meal, we settled into the living room to open gifts. Right there in front of my family and his mom, Steve gave me my very first piece of real gold jewelry. It was a small gold heart on a delicate gold chain. He whispered in my ear, "I think I'm falling in love with you!" Thank goodness for all the commotion with the delightful suspense of unearthing presents, and the rustle of colorful wrapping paper being rolled into balls for the trash. Surely no one heard him. I simply melted in his arms as I sat on his lap waiting for my next package. "Love" is everything I dreamed it would be. And boy did I ever dream a lot. Thank you mom and dad for all your fighting! You taught me how to dream. And now I get to enjoy this moment of having my deepest "darkest hour" dream come true. Thank you too, God. Gosh, I'm only eighteen and I already know that dreams really do come true!

February 19, 1980

I wish that Valentine's Day turned out to be as lovely as Thanksgiving and Christmas. I've been really worried about Mom, and I'm afraid I was preoccupied with worrying about her the evening Steve and I celebrated our first Valentine's Day together. Mom is having a difficult season. Perhaps it's the letdown after all the holidays. I don't know what causes these changes in Mom, but it is just awful to see her this way. Steve has a sister who suffers from depression and he is quite in tuned with Mom's mood swings. He has been sensitive to my feelings, and offers to have our dates at my parent's house so Mom will have some diversion from her own thoughts. Mom likes Steve, and this seems to work out well.

July 5, 1980

After work and weekends, I spend all my time with Steve. We love driving to White Horse Beach, and the long drive is a great chance to talk. Once in a while we go out for dinner at The Mayflower Restaurant. It's right in Plymouth center with all the historical sites. After wrestling with lobster shells, we're rewarded with yummy meat dipped in melted butter. I still haven't learned lobster eating etiquette and we laugh about the way I struggle while we stroll along the pier and watch the fishing boats. Along with his wisecracks about my table manners, he shares his dreams about traveling to California someday.

After such a satisfying weekend, it's so hard to begin the workweek again. I just want to be with him every minute of every day. But I love my job as well. It's intellectually challenging, which I need. It does wonders for my self-esteem. My workload mostly revolves around being the secretary at a physical therapy office, but I am also training to be an assistant for the therapists. I am learning medical terminology and all about the human anatomy. I like what I do and I like the people that I work for. Steve thinks I'm very smart and wonders why I never went to college. I probably should have...

We've been dating for over a year now. At nineteen, I'm still a virgin! And I'm proud of it! I want to be ready and I want us both to care for each other. Steve has not pressured me to sleep with him. I love him for that. He must be interested in me for my personality and intelligence and not just for my body. I know that Steve

Impossible Choices

respects how I feel. I am proud of our relationship. My friends can't believe we haven't done it yet. I don't care, they're not me.

May 26, 1981

Well it happened. Yep, yup! Oh, my God, I just can't believe it! Steve and I slept together. It was wonderful! He was wonderful! I feel wonderful! I've never felt this way before. I've crossed the threshold into womanhood, and that is for sure. Steve told me he loves me! This time it was in private and he didn't say he "THINKS." And I was able to say it back to him. Yes, I am in love! I am bursting with happiness! Nothing else matters in the whole wide world. Not even Mom's spells or Dad's drinking. I'm so much stronger about that now. With Steve at my side, I feel invincible! Over the Memorial Day weekend, we stayed at his parent's cottage at White Horse Beach. We were having an early celebration for our second anniversary. No one knows; it's our secret. Steve told me he loves me and I know I love him. We are great together and everyone thinks we're going to get married. We talk about getting married all the time. We're still pretty young. Steve wants lots of children, too. I'm glad we want the same things. He wants to travel across the country and live in California. He's asked me to go with him. Hmmm... Why not?! I'm twenty years old...

I'm there!

June 23, 1981

I'm traveling to see the country all right. I'm scribbling in my journal in the back seat of Bruce's red Ford Granada rocking down the highway on my way to California! Left two days ago on Sunday, Father's Day. Jeez, didn't mean to drive a knife through Dad's heart by leaving on his special day. It just sort of happened that a U-Haul

Barbara Dooling

truck was available that day. I guess it's not actually a truck; it's more like a bubble that you attach to the top of the car for luggage. I really bawled my eyes out when I left my family on the sidewalk in front of Mom and Dad's house. They had a little cookout for me. Mostly everyone was there to wave good-bye. Lots of hugging and tears. Mom kept making the sign of the cross. Poor Mom and Dad, they were crying to see their baby leaving home. Not only am I leaving, I'm moving out of state! I think I've aged them ten years. God, if they could only pull their shit together! I just can't deal with them sometimes. Why do they waste so many days of their lives being drunk or depressed? I suppose they are chained to their illnesses. What an awful way to live.

This is real living, Route 66... nothing but dust and cows in June...

We're listening to The Rolling Stones blaring out the windows. The plan is to see as many sites in as many states as possible during our fourteen-day journey of "firsts." I don't think this is what Dad had in mind for me when he said, "See the country." I don't imagine he meant move away. And I know he didn't mean move away with a young man. I'm leaving home to move to California with my friends Julie and Bruce, and... Steve! Even though Mom and Dad like Steve, I know they're mortified that we are traveling together and we aren't married. But I think they are more worried that I'll join some cult. They ought to know me by now. I'm not cult material. No way! But I suppose it's a parents right to worry about their children.

When we said our good-byes just a few days ago, everyone was crying. I will be three thousand miles away! I'll miss my family and friends for sure. Sheila isn't coming with us. She's going to be somebody someday. She's going to college. Mary got married this year;

Impossible Choices

I was her maid of honor. I'll miss her terribly. Geno is the only one living at home now. He can play my albums. As for Mom and Dad, I'll miss them, but I won't miss Mom when she's in her wacky state and Dad when he's drunk. For sure!!

My life feels so real now! I can make whatever I want out of it. I'm breaking free! I'm outta here... out of there! Freedom! *Thank God Almighty, I'm free at last*! Gone from Massachusetts to start a brand new awesome life. No more hassles with Mom and Dad's problems. I'm tired of trying to figure them out. I guess I'm running away again. But now that I'm older I can run farther... California is very far! California is perfect! I'm really taking a stand this time. I can't wait to start fresh! I'm going to tread new waters, shake the dust off, and see the world!

June 24, 1981

It is so hot in this car! I'm wilting! My hair is frizzing! I'd like to know whose bright idea it was to cross the United States during the hot summer in a car with no air conditioning. Oh yah, it was mine and Steve's. I guess it could be worse. I could be bouncing around in a covered wagon! The West is so flat. These roads are endless with nothing to look at but farms. They're nice, but the cornfields are a drag after a while. Cows have such a boring life. They don't know it though, so I guess hanging out chewing your cud all day is cool. I can't wait to see Colorado and the Rocky Mountains. What about the Grand Canyon? That's going to be the best! My brother Paul lives in Colorado now. We'll stop to see him, too. What an adventure!

June 26, 1981

Definition of a good day: Driving across country with your friends (and lover) with the wind in your hair and music so loud it

Barbara Dooling

feels like its beating through every inch of your body! Definition of a bad day: Dad drunk and Mom crying. I'm just psyched beyond belief that those days are over! Some people just have no idea what a "bad day" really is! I mean seriously, if I heard one more time from someone that they had the worst day of their life, I'd have screamed! Why do folks even say such bull? Give me a break! Late for a date, stood up, anyway… who cares! Broke a fingernail, ripped your favorite jeans, missed a bus, flunked an exam because you didn't study! Blackheads on your nose, blemishes on your chin, zits on your forehead, zits, zits, zits, are the pits, pits, pits, but surely not the end of the world! Perspective!

June 30, 1981

Well, we're nine days into the trip. Colorado, The Rockies, and The Grand Canyon are definitely all that they're cracked up to be! They're awesome! The Grand Canyon is just amazing. We set up our tent at a campsite in the middle of nowhere. The sun burned our skin, the air was sweltering, and when I went to sit on the hood of the car my fanny got scorched. Once we were settled, we found a scenic viewing area to admire the huge gorge. I'm astonished at how massive it is. The four of us stood speechless, each deep into our own thoughts. The hot wind blew constantly. The valleys of the canyon are many shades of brick red, rusty copper, and cinnamon brown. Part of these extraordinary steep walls are actually red clay. This canyon is truly one of the great wonders of the world. As I stood there, astounded by the miraculous view, something funny happened inside of me. I think it's called being "moved." You know that saying: "I ain't never felt like this before…" that's how I felt. The cloudless blue sky touched the top edges of the cliffs. Except for the wind, the silence was incredible. I might have stayed there all

Impossible Choices

day standing in complete awe, but everyone else was hungry and eager to start supper on the campground grill.

Shortly after we ate, the wind picked up, blowing dirt and dust everywhere. The tent was holding strong as the canvas sides puckered in and out with such force that I thought it might blow away right into the canyon. There was little time to grab our stuff and throw it all into the tent. We didn't know whether to join the luggage in the tent or to flee to the car. We chose the tent and prayed it didn't get swept away with us inside. Dark clouds and heavy rains followed the stormy gusts. Huddled together and out of breath from scrambling about, we all burst into laughter. The storm raged for fifteen minutes, and then... silence again. We stepped out of the tent to find a spectacular double rainbow stretching across the sky! I stared at that prism of transparent colors until it faded. Tears of overwhelming joy filled my eyes. God, it was sensational!

July 1, 1981

Now I'm in San Francisco, California! I'm pen and pool-side at a rinky-dink Motel. The Golden Gate Bridge is awesome! Clouds drifted right through it! We saw Ghiradelli Square, China Town, Fisherman's Wharf, and Lombard Street. I like San Francisco with its Victorian houses painted in pastel colors just for me. The streets here are sloped with very high hills. Tomorrow we'll drive along Highway 1 down to Southern California.

July 2, 1981

I didn't think we could top The Grand Canyon, but The Pacific Coast Highway is darn close! How incredibly beautiful! I keep screaming to Bruce or Steve, "Stop the car! Stop the car!" I've used all my six rolls of film, and had to buy more. Bruce is thoroughly exasperated with me and claims we might as well be in that covered wagon because at the rate we're going, we'll never get to LA! I'm sorry, but I've never seen such amazing scenery. It's real and here right in our country!

First of all, the ocean is truly aqua! I've always admired the midnight blue Atlantic, but this… it's a luscious shade of green and blue—turquoise! And the waves are huge, gigantic! They smash up onto the sheerest cliffs I've ever seen. They strike the rock with such great force, that a vast spray of sunshine sparkles mist shoots into the air in all directions. The noise of these eruptions is a fierce pounding. The wind they create never stops! At each scenic viewing area, after I took a zillion pictures, I stood in utter amazement! Bruce keeps honking the horn and yelling out, "Come on Miss UPI, get off the rocks before I push you over the edge!" He goes insane when I ask him to get out of the car for a group photo! Julie and Steve just laugh at us. My hair is wildly tangled today from nature's blustery gales! Bruce says I look like a maniac and threatens to leave me on the side of the road… no sane driver would pick up such a hitchhiker. Steve says he'd pick me up!

July 3, 1981

Between the scenic viewing stops and my bathroom stops, Bruce is really getting ready to dump me off a cliff! He made me pee outside a few times; Bruce leaned on the horn the whole time just to aggravate me. Everybody's a comedian!

July 4, 1981

Hip, Hip Hurray! We're here in lovely Laguna Beach, California to stay who knows how long! Steve's brother Ed, who lives out here, has already set us up in a three bedroom condo. Our place is

Impossible Choices

very spacious… too bad we don't have any furniture! The grounds are meticulous with the greenest grass as thick as carpeting and the most colorful exotic flowers! Wow! It's even got tennis courts and a pool! Tonight we'll celebrate our arrival with fireworks!

July 11, 1981

Oh no! I'm so bummed! My April Angel's wing was broken in the move! Even beneath all that bubble wrap, the wing shattered into tiny pieces, and I can't really glue it back together! Bummer, Bummer, Bummer!

September 15, 1981

We are settled into our new home! I think Julie and I have done a great job decorating with the bare minimums! We blew up some pictures from our trip, mounted them on colored construction paper, and taped them to the walls. For end-tables and night stands, we used some of our moving boxes and put doilies and table clothes on top. We bought a used refrigerator at a secondhand store in the wrong part of town! Got home and the next day our kitchen was infested with cockroaches! It was so gross! When Steve pulled the frig outside and unscrewed the back grate, zillions of ugly brown roaches with antennae spilled out. They looked like they were waving to us. Oh my God, it was so disgusting! Then we chanced buying a living room set at a yard sale… it's in good shape, except it's pretty dated. It's red and gold crushed velvet! It came with a big ottoman.

To make our place complete, we splurged and got a cute fuzzy kitten! He's orange and white with delicate round ears and tiny paws! We call him TC after the cartoon cat Top Cat! Bruce and TC always fight for the ottoman. Before the evening is over, the kitty is sprawled out and Bruce is left with his feet hanging over the edge! Oh yah, puss-puss got fleas and we had to bomb the house for a second time! I thought everyone was going to kill me cause it was me who wanted the cat! They've been calling my TC: flea bag! King Kitty cat proudly sits and flaunts his fluffy white chest! He is not a flea bag!

October 18, 1981

California is lovely, but the weather is the same every day: sunny and hot, hot and sunny. It hardly ever rains. I'd love to have just one heavy rainstorm. I love a good storm.

The four of us found jobs right away. I'm still working in the medical field and loving it. We eat well, Mom's good cooking rubbed off on me. She'd be proud. With all of us sharing the rent and bills, we are pretty comfortable. Although, when we spend too much money on clothes and parties, there is always macaroni and cheese or French toast for supper.

Laguna Beach is an artist's town. There are many unique shops. The ocean is wild with waves. Biiiiig, GIANT waves. Surfers defy those swells all day, starting at the first crack of dawn. I am not a good swimmer so I mostly sit beachside. The water is much warmer than back east. It is also a lighter green. Instead of catching sunrises on the East Coast, we watch the sun set over the Pacific. Usually it is a huge red ball of fire. The sky turns pink and purple. Steve and I try to go down the beach as often as we can and watch the sunset "show." We are deeply in love. It is so peaceful to walk the beach hand in hand with him. Steve says he cherishes me because I'm so special. He admires my passion for the ocean and nature. We laugh together all the time. He's got dry wit like Bruce and the two feed off each other. But when I need him to be serious, he is! Like

Impossible Choices

when we were back in Massachusetts and he'd see Mom in one of her moods or Dad when he was drunk. Steve always found the right words to make me feel better. He would talk about how great my parents were when they didn't have these problems going on. I'm glad he saw the good in them. Well, now he's taken me away from all that. I'm so happy.

I'm lucky that I was able to get a job at a doctor's office. Got a position assisting for a Pediatrician, and the babies and children love me! I'm in my glory, playing with hand puppets while I try to distract them from the scary man who jabs at their little bodies, sticks a cold metal circle on their tummies and pokes around in their ears. And nothing's worse than having someone force a stick practically down your throat.

Ouch! I got bit on the hand today by a frightened two-year-old boy. I suppose if someone was holding my arms down while a giant in a white coat was coming at me with a pointy needle, I'd defend myself too. All this for a crummy Sesame Street sticker. They ought to have a furry little bunny rabbit for each child to cuddle and play with while the doctor or nurse gives the injections! I mean real live bunnies! That would surely take the kids' minds off the medical stuff. Yah, how come they don't have precious little animals to look at or hold! I suppose it's a health issue... Gosh, it's just too bad cause I'm sure it would work!

December 1, 1981

This is incredible. Bruce has announced to us that he wants to return to Medford for good. It's only been six months, but he's going back home to live. I had a feeling he was homesick, but I didn't imagine he would go back so soon. Bummer. Major bummer! I'll really miss that brat! Who's going to fight with TC? Who will keep the furniture dusted? Who's going to scare the little kids out of the pool and the tennis courts? Who's going to make us laugh? We seemed to be like a family, now it's not going to be the same.

December 22, 1981

Steve and I flew back home for Christmas! Wait a minute, isn't California my home now?

We landed at Logan today. Tons of relatives from both sides met us at the airport. It was so exciting. There were lots of water works! Everyone was crying. I hugged Mom and Dad for such a long time. They look great! Steve's family followed us to Mom and Dad's house for a little welcome home party. Hey, there's snow on the ground! How perfect! A white Christmas. We put up a small tree back at the condo in Laguna… It's not the same feeling without a cold wintry night and snow for Santa! We'll fly back to LA two days after Christmas. I don't even want to think about the sobbing when we depart again!

January 11, 1982

I talk to Mary a lot. She usually calls me on Sundays. Sometimes I call her during the week, especially when I am homesick for family. And boy, do I miss her! She's been keeping me up to date with the goings on with Mom and Dad. I'm grateful Mary lives near enough that she sees them all the time. What a gem Mary is to help take Mom to the doctor's. It's always better to have an extra set of ears when a physician is giving a mini course on medical terminology. From what Mary tells me, Mom is doing much better. She has longer periods of harmony! After all these years of suffering, a doctor has finally diagnosed her with a chemical imbalance. Furthermore, when Mom had a hysterectomy shortly after I was

Impossible Choices

born, she was never given hormone therapy to supplement the immediate loss of estrogen. Without replacing these hormones, Mom experienced major changes like mood swings, migraines, and severe hot flashes. It is no wonder that she had such difficulty with all this going on inside her body. How wonderful it is Mom's getting the help that she needs!

It is awful that she has lost a lot of friends over her illness. These are well-meaning people who just couldn't understand her, and didn't want to take the time to either. I am guilty of the same ignorance! I ran from her, too! My heart aches for my mother's pain and suffering. She is the most beautiful person that I know. Perhaps with her new physician and better medication, Mom will be Mom again... for always.

July 10, 1982

I have been living in California for a year now. I've met some good friends: Christine, Chucky, and Mike. Together with Steve, we've traveled all over this great big state. We've ventured as far north to see Big Bear and Big Sir, the forest area with huge redwood trees... Sausalito... Los Angeles and Hollywood, and as far south as San Diego and Mexico. As much as I have seen, as much as there is still to see, I am homesick for New England. I miss the changing of the four seasons. I miss my family and friends back East. I keep thinking of where I grew up. I think I want to go home. My childhood memories have been flitting through my head a lot lately. For some reason, I can't fight them away today.

There were good times at our house, despite the bad times. I miss cooking with Mom and helping Dad in the garden. Dad knows a lot about flowers and trees. He taught me the names of so many beautiful blossoms and trees. Mom and Dad love nature. I guess

Barbara Dooling

that's why I do. Mom can sit for hours on the beach and watch the ocean. Dad respects all living things, be they plants or critters. I guess that old saying is true… "There's no place like home." Right about now I feel like Dorothy Gale, thankful for these greener pastures that made me appreciate the plush meadows of my own back yard. It's the same way with folks who want to be left alone, and then cry from the loneliness! What's the deal with life? Why do I have this longing for my family today?

I write to Mom and Dad every week, and still call them twice a week. Pacific Bell just loves me! Mom's been telling me that Dad has really been trying to stay sober, and that she too, is doing better. As I sit here rehashing—searching my soul for some answers—I think back to all the challenges Mom and Dad have faced. At times it seemed that they were just existing, going through the motions of day-to-day living. But I now realize that their strong bond of love carried them through. I really want to go back home; I missed so much of my childhood always running to the cemetery or to Sue's house, or tuning out with music up in my room. I want to go home and have a normal day, an ordinary week, a whole year of normal with my family. I really, really want that… so very much. But the only way to get it, is to give all of this up! Leave behind my awesome beach and freedom along with my new identity. California is a paradise. I have everything I've ever dreamed of. A free spirit, living it up on the beaches of California with great friends and a guy that I love? This is all true.

But lately I've been feeling that what I really want is a family to call my very own. I must really want it a lot because today I am thinking that I want it more than this spectacular California seaside. Perhaps that's why I'm feeling so blue today. I want to be a mother, and have a little girl at my side just as I was with my own mother.

Impossible Choices

When I talk to Mom and Dad, I can tell they really miss me. I miss them, too. I need one of my dad's big hugs. I am thinking maybe I'm done with this California adventure. Oh, what should I do? I need to steal away to the beach, and go talk to my ocean to figure this out. What about Steve? Will he want to go back to Boston? I hope so.

July 17, 1982

Steve and I walked along Laguna Beach tonight. The sunset was exceptionally beautiful. He commented that the sun was brilliant and the sky was splashed with vibrant colors. He truly loves living in California; this I know. He is very happy. I told him that I wanted to go back home. As I spoke, I cried because I knew that Steve wanted to stay. I sobbed on his shoulder and asked him what we were going to do. He actually walked away from me. I sat on the beach alone while Steve collected his thoughts. I wondered what decision he would make. I wondered if maybe he would ask me to marry him so that I would stay. I thought about what I would do if he did not ask me to marry him.

After a long while, he walked back to where I was sitting. He had tears in his eyes. I have never seen a man cry before except for my dad when Mom was sick. I remember Dad saying that it was good for a man to cry. That it meant he was sensitive. Steve wasn't just crying, he was trembling, even though the evening was warm. He had made his decision and I feared it was to break up with me. (I lacked confidence in this younger relationship.) But Steve said he did not want to lose me. He told me that he would move back to Boston with me. We hugged and kissed. Both of us were crying. We sat quietly until the sun finally went down behind the horizon.

Barbara Dooling

August 1, 1982

We are on the plane going back home… for good. Bruce has been gone for eight months, and Julie is staying on in California. Bruce is picking us up at the airport. Can't wait to see him; I've missed him so much. Julie took us to LAX. We cried like babies when we said our good-byes. I've gotten really close to Julie since our trip out here. I wish she was going back home, too.

I'm really going home. We're really going home. Together. Steve and I are leaving California together! I can't wait to see everyone again. Mary is pregnant! She's asked me to be the baby's godmother! Geno is engaged! He and his fiancé Karen have asked me to be in their wedding! Kenny has moved to Newport, Rhode Island. He's invited me to see the Newport mansions and the lovely beaches. Russ and Ann have moved to Dedham. I'll get to see my two nieces, Kim and Kerry. Sheila has graduated from Boston College with honors. She's so smart. I even can't wait to see Steve's family. During the four years we've been dating, I have grown very fond of his whole family especially Elli. She is so dear to me. I love all of his four sisters and his two brothers and his dad. We're going to see everyone again!

April 24, 1983

Sitting on my old bed in my old room. Just celebrated my twenty-second birthday, and yep, I'm back at Mom and Dad's—for now anyway. Steve and I didn't have any money when we first got back from California. Plus, I decided it wasn't a good idea for us to live together here right under our parent's noses. I don't know, I just felt funny about it. Steve was bummed out, but he agreed with me. I think he was more worried about what my parents thought than his own. We have settled into our old routines of working and

Impossible Choices

dating. Something is wrong with Steve, though. I just know it. He is different since we've been back. He does not seem happy.

May 6, 1983

I'm devastated! Tonight Steve told me that he wants to go back to California. He never mentioned us getting married. I won't give him an ultimatum, but I'm not going back to California unless we get married. I didn't tell him this. I want him to ask me to marry him because he wants to, not because I've pushed him into it. I don't think he is ready to get married, and I'm through playing house with him. I need a family to call my own. If we were to marry, Steve and I would make our own family. I can't go back with him. I just can't. How will I let him leave me though? I love him. What's going to happen to us? I am so torn between the love in my heart and the awareness in my brain. Some of my friends say that they could never let him go. Steve and I want different things right now. I must give him this space to find what he wants. And I must think about my own needs. I have to face reality… if he didn't want to lose me, wouldn't he ask me to marry him and to move back to California with him? I've told him how I feel. Now it's up to him to make his choice. I have to let him go and find out what he really wants. But what if I lose him forever?

May 13, 1983

Sat in Steve's car for such a long time tonight talking about the future. What future? His? Mine? Ours? He keeps saying that he wants us to be together, yet there is no mention of marriage. Haven't we been dating long enough? Four years. What's he waiting for? If I go back to California with him, it's going to be the same as it was before. We'd be living together biding time. I know him well enough, he knows me. Maybe we are too young. I know that's why he's dragging his feet. He's only twenty-four. What do I expect? I wish we could stay here for a couple more years, get married, then move out West. Steve is just so restless. He's got to go now. Now is too soon to tie the knot and I can't just keep living with him. So now what?

May 16, 1983

More thinking. Lots more agonizing. I even went to Plymouth over the weekend to be alone with my thoughts. I sat by myself on the beach for the whole afternoon. Actually, I wasn't totally alone. A million memories were there too. As the spring breeze whisked through my hair, I stared at the whitecaps, wishing for some answers. I've been happy with Steve. So what is my problem? The flashbacks tug at my heart, and reality pulls me in another direction. I feel that I must let Steve go—for now. He must be free to make his move, and I need to allow myself to find out a painful truth. I know that he loves me; I just don't know if he loves me enough to spend the rest of his life with me. This moment will reveal everything that I need to know. I'm not sure how I shall bare this, but it has to be done for my own good.

May 29, 1983

He left today; I've been crying ever since. All I have now are "Photographs and Memories" like the song by Jim Croce. My heart is broken. I feel sick inside. He begged me to go back to California with him and I said no. What have I done? What am I going to do without him? I'm shattered! Maybe I should have gone. Oh, I just don't know. My heart is telling me that I should have gone, but my head is saying if he really wanted me, we would have gotten

Impossible Choices

engaged. There had to be some promise... some commitment for the future. Oh, Steve, why didn't you ask me to marry you? I still don't understand. We used to talk about marriage all the time. I'm plain miserable. I'm going to lose him; I just know it. We'll probably never see each other again. Four long years of loving and laughing. Everyone always said we were the perfect couple. Look at us now. Me and my damn values. Me and my damn dreams. Now I have to live with my choice.

His family went to the airport with us to say their good-byes. They all watched as we embraced... I softly kissed his lips and they were wet with his tears. Steve whispered, "I love you, Barb. I love you, Kiddo." I couldn't even get the words out. I sobbed, "I love you, too." And then I turned around. I walked right out of that airport and never looked back. I cried the whole way home. I am crying now as I write this. What on earth have I done? There goes my Little House on The Prairie. Oh, my house in the country will never be built. I'll never have that house full of kids like The Walton's.

January 18, 1984

It's been almost eight months since Steve left Boston. I've taken a new position with a physical therapy practice. I like it very much and the people I work with are great! Steve and I continue to write to each other, although we are both dating other people. A long distance romance is just that—distant. Steve asked me to visit him in California. He said he would pay for my airfare. I'm considering it; I just don't know.

I've been seeing this guy Ed. He's gorgeous. I'd even say neck-and-neck with Steve, except Ed is taller and even more muscular. Ed jogs and works out at the gym everyday. He's got biceps that look like they've been stuffed with cold playdough. He used to play football in college; now he coaches. His neck is massive and his abdomen solid muscle. His thick jet black hair and green eyes are breathtaking! But I don't love Ed. He's not as sensitive and caring as Steve. He doesn't caress me or really try to please me by doing something nice and thoughtful like cooking dinner or helping me fix my car. I think he's more into his looks than he is into me. I think I'm jealous of his running schedule. Snow, rain, or shine, the man is pounding the streets in a sweat suit. He is obsessed, even in a storm he has to run. When we lounge around on the couch, he'd rather be watching his favorite football team steal a few yards than make way for a kiss from me. I've caught him sizing up other women when we're out at a restaurant. I wouldn't mind, even I like to look, but it's the way he does it that makes me feel uncomfortable. It's like, "would you like me to leave so you can go ask her out?" My self-esteem crumbles when he practically drools over some blond. I don't need that! I joke with him about it. I tell him that I could never have a serious relationship with him.

February 14, 1984

I am Valentine-less! I called Steve tonight. I had decided to take him up on his offer of a spontaneous visit... that is until he asked me to stay with Julie. I get it now; he doesn't want to jeopardize his new relationship. I don't think this is going to work out too well. Nope, I'm not hiding out at Julie's apartment. He wants his cake and to eat it too. He can't have both. At least not with me. I still love him. I love him too much to share him. This is going to be difficult. Well, I'm twenty-two years old, and I've already lived through the hardest part of this saga—I really can do this. I can do this. I can tell him "no"...

But maybe I should go. Both Sheila and Julie want me to see

Impossible Choices

him—to fight for him. They think that once he sees me again, he'll come running back to me. How can I have a good time when this other woman exists in his heart enough to ask me not to stay with him? Well, I just won't do it! I won't stay at Julie's apartment. I told him exactly that. I've made my choice—hard as it is. This was the right decision. Although my heart is in torment, my mind is at peace.

My first love and I made a lot of lovers' promises that day he left Boston. For a while we wrote to each other, and I kept in touch with his family. Now I have to cut the cord, and save my tender, loving memories. I've grown into a different woman since my love affair with Steve. I am more confident and I know what I want out of a relationship. I do not regret a single day that I spent with that man. Nor do I regret my decision to stay home. I'll probably never see him again. This is hard; life is hard. I am learning that real life is not about fairytale endings, but rather managing how to handle the real ending. Happily ever after is about finding a way to be happy after the tale fades. Turned out it wasn't much of a nice Valentine's Day, but it was a growth moment, so the day wasn't a total loss.

May 10, 1984

So, I am alone! Yep, me, myself, and I. I have no boyfriend. At all. But I do have peace of mind. Now that's an accomplishment! Despite my pride, I do have a heavy heart. Can one possibly have both—a clear mind and a light heart? Sometimes there has to be a tradeoff. It's like the heart can be so full of joy and love that it clouds the mind—blocks reality. I could have a boyfriend right now, but I would not be true to myself. It can be difficult to reason with yourself because you keep wanting to have both—to have it all! I am learning that when you can't have everything, there has to be a compromise. You sometimes have to settle for the tradeoff, and be happy with that. Or else—what else? What's the other option? Oh yah... misery.

I've dated several men since my breakup with Steve. I don't feel the same about them as I did with him. But I'm enjoying my life. I don't mind not having a steady boyfriend. Since I've turned twenty-three, I'm happy with me. Mom and Dad are doing a little bit better. Dad still drinks, but not as often, or as much. Mom has found a good psychiatrist who has put her on antidepressant medication that seems to be working for now. I love my new job. I'm continuing to learn a lot about the medical field. I'm always asking lots of questions. In addition to managing the physical therapy practice, I have been learning to assist the therapists. I guess you could say I do it all. Each day that passes, I feel better about the breakup. I'm glad I was strong enough to think of myself. I heard that he married the woman he was dating. Wow, that was fast. So you see, if he really wanted to marry me, he would have asked me. He is obviously capable of getting married! Marriage wasn't the conflict, like I had assumed. The issue was me. Ouch, that hurts!

I wish him happiness. I have no regrets about our relationship. He'll always be my first love. We had some wonderful times together. It was a beautiful, wonderful us! We parted the best of friends. I'm glad that I'll always be able to look back on that part of my life with great satisfaction. Our relationship was good. We simply grew apart. We wanted different things in the end. He'll be in my heart for a long time, but it's not the same feeling now. I am proud of myself for standing my ground. I will find the right man for me. All good things come to those that wait, right?

Impossible Choices

June 13, 1984

I've got a crush on a cute guy at work. His name is Jack and he's one of the physical therapists. Me thinks he has the hots for yours truly, too. Today, he joked with me by calling from one of the internal phone lines. He pretended to be a patient trying to book an appointment for "physical" therapy wanting a massage and a few other interesting things. I explained to the phony patient that these services were not provided at this particular practice. It took me a moment, but I recognized Jack's voice and called him a Jerk. He sometimes flies a paper airplane into my office with a funny message. I seem to get lots of attention from him and he's always offering to make runs to the cafeteria to pick up my lunch or an afternoon cup of tea. Once in a while he'll bring back a treat like a chocolate chip cookie. We both wish that we didn't work together, but there is little chance either of us will be changing jobs in the near future. I'm pretty certain that I don't want to take things an inch further because I don't want any office politics to ruin my reputation… People love their gossip.

December 15, 1984

The company Christmas party was quite the challenge! After a couple of drinks, Jack and I danced… "cheek to cheek" as they say. He secretly asked me to meet him at his car afterwards. I did. We exchanged a quick kiss good-bye. It could have gone further, but I got hold of my senses and told Jack that although I would love to date him, I didn't think it was a good idea while we are still working together. A secret fling is out of the question for me. I made this perfectly clear. I did not give in to his sad eyes. I went straight home (with a heavy heart). Now that's strength!

Barbara Dooling

February 14, 1985
Jack slipped me a cute Valentine's Day card. He gets an "A" for effort!

July 13, 1985
Guess where I am? Sheila, Bruce, Dave (Bruce's friend), and I jetted off to New York City for the weekend! I've known Dave through Bruce for a few years now. What a cutie! But… he's spoken for. Just my luck. We have become good friends and this weekend will be difficult to mind my manners since he didn't bring the flame. I can surely look, though!

Dave is such a sweetheart. He's caring, funny, and lovable. Why is he taken? Ugh! He's short, dark, and handsome! And staying in the same hotel suite with me! I'm like a cat in heat. I don't think Dave has a clue that I like him. And if you ask me, I think Sheila's heart is throbbing, too. Yah, she acts as stupid as me around Dave. Last night we went to a nightclub and kicked up our heals dancing. David dances like no other guy I know. He's fantastic. Sheila and I stayed out on the parquet floor song after song after song. Bruce pooped out, but we danced for so long that our hair was soaking. I've been heated up all weekend. The temperature reached a hundred and nine degrees yesterday. Imagine how sweltering this city is in the middle of a heat wave? Never mind the fact that I'm ablaze with hormones. This infatuation is as difficult as the one I've got with Jack. What is it? Jeez, I'd better get back on the subject of Broadway, Radio City, Tavern on the Green, The Statue of Liberty, The Empire State Building! All of which we have already seen! Tomorrow we go for brunch before our flight back to Boston.

Impossible Choices

August 5, 1985

I just can't believe it... Jack is not only leaving the physical therapy rehab, he's moving to Chicago! He is going back to school to become a doctor. The announcement was a shock! He will be gone by September. I'm happy for him and all, except that we still can't pursue a relationship. He invited me to his apartment—not sure for what. No way am I going to start anything now with him leaving in two weeks. I told him that I'd write to him. We shall see where the heck this goes.

November 14, 1985

Julie is still living in California. We write and chat by phone, and she tells me all about her lifestyle on the West Coast. At twenty-four, I'm here in New England where I belong—with my family. At times, I do think about my adventure out West, especially when a song comes on the radio like *California Dreamin'* by The Mamas and The Papas, or *Surfer Girl* by The Beach Boys. But Mom and Dad are doing well these days, and I am happy to be here with them. I am grateful for their commitment to each other and to the family unit. I am looking forward to the upcoming holidays with them. I can only imagine their past struggles. It is good to see them enjoying their children and grandchildren. This is what I had prayed for so many years ago. Thank you, God, for giving my parents back to me. I love them so!

July 13, 1986

Today was an eventful day: bought my first brand new car, moved into an apartment with Bruce, and went to the Moody Blue's concert. I'm sitting in our empty living room on a lounge chair. We ordered a new set, a couch, love seat and chair. It won't be delivered until next week. Bruce and I are very good friends, our relationship is strictly platonic. He came with me to pick out my blue, four- door Chevy Cavalier, and quite unexpectedly wound up buying the same car in red. That salesman was in his glory! The concert was great, except it poured rain and it was outdoors! For such a busy day, I'm making my entry short. Have to get up tomorrow and unpack lots of boxes. It's late... too late to think and write any more.

October 24, 1986

I just got back from a mini vacation in Colorado. Visited Paul and Maureen; their first baby Stephany was christened. She's just precious and she is so tiny with the darkest hair. It was a pleasant trip, but after seeing that new little family, I yearn to have my own baby. I continue to take pleasure in spending as much time as possible with all my nieces and nephews. At least they fill the void in my heart. Wow, I'm twenty-five and there's no man in sight. I am thankful for my family.

November 30, 1986

Jack came home for Thanksgiving last week and I invited him to one of my favorite places—Newport. He accepted; I was really nervous, but excited. We'd finally be able to date.

I picked him up at the airport and we headed down 95 for what I envisioned would be an electric weekend. We had a sensational ride chatting nonstop the entire way. Our day was filled with new romance of holding hands and stealing kisses. I showed him some of the sites around Newport: the scenic waterfront, unique shops, and purgatory chasm, which is a big natural gorge. The ocean thrusts its way into the rift making enormous splashes into the air. We even took in a mansion—The Breakers. I couldn't believe that I

Impossible Choices

was quite possibly feeling the same way as I did with Steve. It was wonderful and thrilling all over again! That night we shared pleasant conversation and a lovely dinner at The White Horse Tavern, a quaint Victorian restaurant. After dinner we danced for hours at The Clark Cook House, another picturesque restaurant and nightclub. What a fine evening! We ended up alone at Kenny's house. Then the night turned sour. I just couldn't believe it! Jack wanted to go to bed with me and I said no. Ugh... why did I say no? My heart and hormones were definitely ready—Nope! Nope! Nope! When I stop and think about it, my head is attached to this body. Yah, the heart and head are both part of me. So I did the right thing for me, and that matters. I'd rather do this and have it be perceived as the wrong thing by him, than the other way around.

I tried to explain myself, but his ears were blocked. I was feeling like we needed more time together as a couple. I was feeling that "I" needed more time. I wasn't ready. I wanted it to be right and I definitely wasn't comfortable yet. My opinion was that Jack was going back to school in just a week. We hadn't even been dating. His opinion was that we had been conversing even if it was by mail. He thought since I invited him away for the weekend, it was assumed that we would sleep together. Oh My God! How naive I am!

We slept in separate rooms and in the morning, we went home. It was a very different ride back. Except for the songs on the radio, the car was silent. There was no fun weekend to continue. I dropped him off and that was good-bye. I am flabbergasted. I keep trying to figure things out. I know that I made the right choice. If he's going to drop me just because I wasn't ready to sleep with him, then he's not actually worthy of me. Really though, we could have been a good couple, and it's too bad that he didn't give me a chance. Who knows what the rest of the weekend would have brought. I think he jumped the gun. I keep coming up with the fact that evidentially Jack did not really respect me and how I felt. So it was just as well that we never had a relationship. I believe it's his loss and I am sorry that we couldn't have at least parted friends. He was so angry.

Well, at least I've learned something from this. I now know what type of man I don't want, which makes me realize what man I do want! I want a man who will be understanding and compassionate. I want a partner that I can communicate with… who's going to listen. I want us to be able to work things out and compromise. Support and caring should be mutual.

August 21, 1987

Sowing my wild oats. Sheila, Bruce and I go to Kenny's in Newport twice a month. I'm at Gooseberry Beach in Newport right now. There are cliffs and rocks all over the beaches in Rhode Island. The ocean rushes against the rocky coast with each wave spraying salty mist into the air. I'd love to have a house on the ocean. I'd love to have a house period. All in good time I suppose. For now, I'll settle for Kenny's house. It's got a great view of the ocean and the Jamestown Bridge—The Diamond Necklace, (that's what the Newporters call it when it's all lit up). The lights sure do shimmer like diamonds.

On Sunday mornings, we sun ourselves on the roof deck while sipping mimosas. This is of course after a weekend of fun and excitement. We kick up our heals dancing in the nightclubs. During the daytime, we hit the shops and wind up at The Black Peal or some other fine restaurant for clam chowder and appetizers. For dinner, we either cook on the grill at Kenny's, or we head out to a restaurant again. The Cliff Walk Manor is our favorite. It's also a

Impossible Choices

hotel. A while back, we celebrated Newport living at that restaurant with lobster and champagne. We were in such high spirits that night that we decided to rent rooms in this mansion. I think if the building had been for sale, we would have bought it! We were out of control! We had adjoining rooms with ocean views.

Another favorite Newport activity is going to Sunday Brunch at The Inn at Castle Hill. It's such a lovely spot located on a big cliff overlooking the ocean. We walk around the grounds or sit for hours, just soaking up that marvelous view. What a life!

June 25, 1988

Still doing the dating scene. Twenty-seven, still haven't met Mr. Right-For-Me. Having a great time looking though. Wow, according to my childhood dreams, I was supposed to be married by now, maybe even with a couple of kids. But I don't want to choose Mr. Available just because the time is right. There is more to life than finding a husband. It's amazing how girls grow up with this fantasy of their prince from the moment they first read Cinderella. Who wouldn't want to be carried off in a carriage with white horses? It sounds enchanting! One of the orthopedic doctors from work and her husband had a big bash today. It was their annual fund-raiser; the contributions are donated to burn victims. The husband Bobby had a bad accident a number of years ago and was horribly burned in a fire at his auto body shop. So they've been hosting an annual gathering at their home each June for the past five years that I know of. It's an over-the-top affair just like a huge wedding reception. I like going for the fine food and live band entertainment. I am usually on the prowl for a doctor, anesthesiologist… Some wonderful man to sweep me off my feet. Didn't find him today, but it was sensational just the same. The one great thing about not having a boyfriend is that I've developed many friendships that I never would have otherwise. I had a great time today socializing with all my friends—thankful for the opportunity to fill my heart's scrapbook with such fun memories. I saw one couple sitting poolside, and all they did was bicker at each other. I'm not sure who they were, but it wasn't the time or place for fighting. I marched myself as far away from them as I could! Thank goodness I don't have those sorts of memories. Mine are warm with sunshine and splendor, and I'll cherish them for all the years to come!

December 31, 1989

WOW! This year is going out with a lot of news! There were three births with three Christenings, another trip to Colorado, a vacation down the cape, a ninetieth birthday, a forty-fifth wedding anniversary, Julie's return home from California (FOREVER), and my tenth high school reunion! Baby Michael is Geno and Karen's third son, Marissa—Paul and Maureen's second daughter, and Kenny Jr. is who other than Kenny's first! I attended all the Christenings including the Baptism of sweet Marissa which took place in June. In August, I had the pleasure of taking my two oldest nieces Kim and Kerry and a group of their friends down to Falmouth. I was the lone chaperone with this teenage clan. What a scream—literally! Between the music and the girls, I'm not sure who was louder! All I kept telling my nieces was that their father was going to kill me. But Russ and Ann didn't have to worry—not really. I kept everything under control (relatively speaking of course).

In October, Nana turned ninety. She's Dad's mother. This ancient woman still has natural black hair with only streaks of gray. She's got the smoothest skin, and all her faculties. She's amazing! Just one week later, we celebrated Mom and Dad's forty-fifth at a lovely

Impossible Choices

Restaurant with everyone except Paul and Maureen and my spouse who I haven't met yet. Yep, I was the odd ball at the table—didn't even have a date. But I took all the pictures of each couple.

Julie has moved back East after nine years in California. I only went out to visit her once during that whole time, (she may have traveled home for the holidays once or twice), but that's it. I've missed her and I'm glad she is home to stay.

My tenth year high school reunion was the last big event. It was pleasant enough. Hmmm... I turned twenty-eight this year. Seeing all my old friends made for an interesting evening. I had a few laughs, envied the girls who were married or pregnant, marveled at those who excelled in their careers, and silently thanked God I wasn't one of the divorced crowd. I had a warm glow all night, excited to think that I still had all this in front of me, just like the day I graduated. I hadn't aged a day. Forever young... That's me, Miss Forever Young... and wide-eyed, hopeful, and forever on the verge of the "Best is yet to come." I think my friends were a little envious of my green pastures sprawled out before me, despite the fact that we're the same age. One day, it will be me who is married and pregnant! Yep, all these people are married and that's great, but their weddings are all behind them, and I still have mine to look forward to. Even better is that I have not married the wrong person just for the sake of it, just so I could show up at my ten year reunion married. I'm still "free at last!" I'm happy with all my choices. I'm proud to be me. I'm okay with where I am going; my career is satisfying and I'm content with just me. WAHOO!

August 25, 1990

I've met some very nice men. Let's see: There's been Dave who likes to go to concerts. We went to see the Alman Brother's togeth-

Barbara Dooling

er. Concerts are super, but you can't talk and get to know someone with deafening music blasting. A lot of guys like to take me to the movies. But I'd rather go on a picnic and sit by the Charles River in Boston. I'd like to go roller-skating along the river, something like that. What about the beach? That would be a super date! Pack up a blanket and some lunch. Maybe a little Vino and cheese. Take along a kite to soar and run with. On a date like that, at least you can talk and share dreams. Some men don't like to get into heavy conversation. I have found these are men who are just not looking for a serious relationship. Many are afraid of commitment.

And let's see... there was Mike... so sweet... but... BUT... there is a very big BUT. Our relationship was just missing that spark. At least for me anyway. It is difficult not to compare men to Steve. I've got to stop doing that. He was my first love, and he'll always have that spot in my heart. It's been seven years, and Steve still has a piece of my spirit, whether he knows it or not. Suppose that's a good thing to be able to look back with fond memories. Some beautiful fine day my new man will sweep me off my feet. I'm willing to wait because I'm not going to settle for less than wonderful.

Everyone is married now except me. Every family has one—the unmarried aunt. But I have lots of nieces and nephews now to dote over. I have been traveling just like I always wanted to do. Seems I've been to Florida at least half a dozen times. I've visited Paul and Maureen out in Colorado twice, and I've been to Canada—Nova Scotia. I've taken great pleasure on these trips and I'm saving for the next one. I want to see Europe. Paris would be heavenly. But is that a place for lovers? I may have to wait on that.

March 15, 1991

Aaahhh... the Caribbean Beach Resort in Disney World, Florida.

Impossible Choices

Such a great hotel right on Disney property. I've tagged along as Bruce's guest on his vacation with his entire family. It's been the grandest! Bruce cracks me up. Everyone should have a Bruce in their life. What a comedian! He likes to joke with me about finding my prince charming. He says I'm full of dreams. Yes, I am! He tells me I better hurry up or they'll be wheeling me down the aisle with gray hair. I'm only twenty-eight. I'm not that old or am I? So much for my blueprint life—being married by now. The Man Upstairs must have someone very special in mind just for me... patience...

Disney World has got to be the most magical place there is! I just love Disney! All the theme parks are sensational, but my very favorite has to be Magic Kingdom. We visited this park today. I'm still smiling! Seeing all those children sparkling with delight makes me want to cry. I did cry. Bruce of course calls me "water works." I forced Bruce to go on It's a Small World. That ride is a must! I was singing the Small World song in the long line and all through the entire ride. He was ready to cart me off to one of those countries.

Seeing all the people here in Disney gets me to thinking again that I'd sure like to have one of those All American families. Especially the young couples who are on their honeymoon and people with their small children, some are pregnant expecting another child. I have enjoyed the company of Bruce and his family, but I sure do wish I had one of those families of my own.

April 28, 1991

The Big 30! Mary threw a surprise birthday party at the VFW Hall in Dedham. April Angel adorned the top of my cake! She didn't forget to invite my Angel. My lovely Angel is getting so old. She's got that broken wing, has more chips, and her colors are more faded. Nevertheless, she still brightens my spirit. Whenever I look at her,

Barbara Dooling

it's like she's smiling at me. She may have a damaged wing, but her grin makes me soar. Who needs wings to fly? I'm happy and that says everything. I don't mind turning thirty. I love my life and all my friends and relatives who gave me such a warm welcome to my thirties. There was no man at my side for the "swearing in," ... But I hardly noticed I was having so much fun. Mary had decorated with the help of Sheila and Bruce. She certainly nailed every detail: from colorful streamers to the delicate yellow roses for centerpieces. She even did most of the cooking, and there was enough food to feed the town of Dedham. A DJ played hit songs from the seventies and eighties, which sure brought back some amusing memories. Geno requested *Birthday* by the Beatles! That was the best! I've come a long way with my dancing since that night in Bermuda. Bruce calls me "Ginger" after Ginger Rogers! The grand finalé was the presentation of gag gifts: a bottle of old-lady vitamins, denture tablets, a box of adult diapers, and some hair coloring. Nice friends, huh?

Mom and Dad were there, and of course beaming with pride. I think they imagine that I'm twenty—not thirty (I guess it's that not-being-married thing again). I'll always be their baby! Dad just keeps saying, "You're how old? Oh my gosh!" Mom repeats, "Thirty?" and then makes the sign of the cross. They're so cute. She pinched my cheeks and said, "*Bella, Bella. Que facha Bella.*" If I've spelled this correctly, that's beautiful, beautiful, what a beautiful face! Thanks Mom! She and all my aunts have a habit of squeezing and pinching the cheeks of every child on the planet. They're so cute! Kenny does it to me, too, and still calls me his little Coochie Kapooli! To this day! At least Ken's pinches don't hurt as much. Italian moms and aunts can leave bruises! By today's standards, that's child abuse!

Sure was pleasant having my real parents at my party instead of the impostors. (I won't even go there because the folks are doing

Impossible Choices

so well, and that's all I want to think about.) Mom and Dad danced up a storm tonight, even to the pop music. In their day, they used to clear the floor! People would form a circle just to watch them Polka! Dad would yell out whoops and hollers while he swung Mom around like a rag doll. When I have witnessed this "quickstep," I've noticed that they strut about as if they were one. Every time I tried to dance with Dad tonight, he said I kept fighting him for the lead. He pleaded, "Follow me! Please follow me." But I strained instead of loosening up! It was me and him all over all right, only I was so dizzy from him twirling me, and out of breath from skipping up and down the length of that dance floor, that I got a pain in my right side and had to sit down. And I'm how old? And Dad and Mom are what…seventy-three and sixty-eight? Who are the seniors here? Then Mom threw some salt in the wound and said "In my hay day, I could really cut a rug. I danced from the waltz to the Charleston. Then the jitter bug became the craze." Dad can't jitter bug, but Mom tried to teach me tonight! I just love it. What a fun dance. I kept stepping on her toes and banging into her. By late evening, we tried it once more and I think I've got it! I want to learn all of these dips, steps, and twirls!

The night ended too quickly and now I'm sitting in the living room with opened presents and saved bows. Besides the funny gifts, I got candles, clothes, frames, and all sorts of wonderful things. Wow, am I really thirty?! Seems like I just graduated from High School. What happened to twenty? Oh yah, I was gallivanting the countryside. I don't regret a single day, especially my first love. I've never seen or heard from dear Steve again—it's been eight years. I wonder how he is. I wonder how he's aging, ha ha.

Well, I'm happy with me so far. I can't help but wonder what my future holds. I know that I want to keep traveling. I'm still saving for my big trip to Paris. Sheila wants to go, too. Her friend from college wants to join us to make a traveling trio. Marlene was a Nanny for a family in Paris for over a year. She'd be a great person to travel with since she speaks French very well. Maybe we'll go next year. It seems so far away, but the funds are just not there. Between rent and car payments, there's little money left over for savings. I'll get there though; I'm determined!

June 30, 1992

I've left my job at the physical therapy office. Wow, I've been with them for five years, and in this specialty for nine. It was a sad day. I really enjoyed working for this group, but the practice moved to Medfield—too far of a commute. Started managing an Internal Medicine practice with two physicians. It's a whole new language... a much broader range of medicine, but I love it! I'm learning so much, and the doctors appreciate my enthusiasm. Helping people when they're sick is very rewarding for me. I've held the hands of many patients, young and old. It's a great feeling. My place is definitely in the medical field.

Administration is more challenging than ever before with HMO's taking over the insurance companies. The two female doctors who I work for are PCPs—Primary Care Physicians. Patients have to choose a PCP who will manage his or her health care by issuing a paper referral form, only when medically necessary, to another specialty physician, such as an orthopedic. The referral has an actual number assigned to it along with the number of visits a patient can see another doctor. The majority of a patient's medical needs will always begin with seeing their PCP. It is up to the PCP and the HMO to refer patients accordingly when there is a diagnosis that the PCP is unsure of or doesn't particularly handle. I'll say

Impossible Choices

one thing, it has created much havoc over the last few years because people are used to going to a doctor of their choice. When they have a skin problem they call a dermatologist; a female disorder, it's a gynecologist; an eye disease, an ophthalmologist, and so forth.

The new way of medicine is the patient must see the PCP first, and can no longer elect a doctor without getting prior authorization. And sometimes there are even restrictions as to what "referral circle" or "Network" the PCP is with. This would be the actual hospital they are affiliated with. Also, a sub-specialist such as a psychiatrist, must belong to this insurance organization. Members of a particular insurance company must follow these guidelines to receive the maximum benefits they are allowed. If they choose to go out of network—out of the area that their PCP is located—the benefits are reduced. If they forget to call their PCP for that paper referral, same deal. Worst of all, some companies won't even pay the claim if the referral is missing. Patients are then liable to get a bill from the specialist which creates more calls to PCP, HMOs, and a particular doc who doesn't get paid. It's amazing doctors don't seem to be practicing medicine alone, now they have to concern themselves with all this referring, or if they are a specialist, they must ensure that a referral number is in place or they don't get paid for their services. I see it as a lot of paper pushing amidst the usual hectic day. This has created more demands on everyone in the office as well as overloaded the already overloaded schedule. Patients are required to follow their insurance companies conformities according to these new regulations but they get so confused, especially the elderly.

Folks are afraid of change. The adjustments have been slow, but the way I understand it, the idea is supposed to be cost effective for everyone: PCP, insurance agencies, and patient. I also believe that the PCP gets a certain percentage of the savings back, which is called "Take backs" at the end of the year if they follow the referral system. It's kind of like a rebate. Even though some insurance companies have changed their system over to electronic referrals, there is still a ton of paperwork involved, and PCP's are hiring a separate person just to handle these referrals and insurance issues. There are different rules for each insurance… and everyone knows how many health insurance companies are out there. So that's a lot of things to remember, What is standard for one company, is a separate regulation for another. It's hard to keep up! Wish there was some uniform practice to simplify things.

All this going on among the day-to-day emergencies and patient triage. Where I work, I do it all! Referrals, Urgent Care coordination, billing, balancing monthly reports (that's accounts receivable and payable), claims submission, phoning prescriptions, surgical scheduling, instructing pre-op preparations, hospitalizations, staff supervising, (including hiring, firing, training)…ahmm let's see, what else? Payroll, payroll taxes, directing staff meetings, covering secretaries and medical assistants/technicians during their absence, attending workshops and seminars to keep up with the ever changing medical field, and being primary support to physicians! It's all called managing daily operations in a multiple physician practice!

Today was the day of days! Our front desk receptionist and the medical assistant were both out sick at the same time! Of course it's month-end and I was trying to focus on closing reports. I had to drop everything and literally run back and forth like a polar bear pacing in a cage! …Clean examining rooms, maintain patient flow by getting them to change into gowns, weigh them, take medical history for new patients, dipstick urine and record results, chart

Impossible Choices

blood pressure results, and spin and package tubes of blood to prepare for lab pick up. All this in between answering a multi phone line, collecting co-payments, scheduling appointments! The only thing I didn't accomplish was juggling dynamite sticks for those frustrated patients in the waiting room. HMMM... no problem. I'm sure I could have managed that too if anyone had asked. I feel like I won the Olympic gold medal. I never lost my cool! I was as kind and keen with those patients, and courteous and contributory to both doctors as if it was an ordinary day. In fact I'm so well-trained at overloaded days that surely God must have some really big future plans for me that involve lots of intense strategizing. Seems to me I'm able to work pretty well under pressure. These unbalanced routines happen quite frequently with a smaller practice. There are not a lot of employees here like at a hospital where coworkers can rotate jobs. If you're going to be a team player, you have to be a sport! See? The day of days. I'm tired writing about it let alone living it.

July 18, 1992

Oh Dear, what dismay! Went on a blind date tonight... another frog passing himself off as a prince! One of the girls from work fixed me up with this "Really cute, soooo nice, really wonderful guy." Okay, he was a little bit cute, somewhat nice... but not at all wonderful! His efforts to be polite were a bit much—obvious and forced. He picked me up at 7:00, and by 7:45 I was calling him "the tour guide." He led me by the arm all night. Every time I got up to go to the ladies room, he escorted me, putting his hand around my waist and pushing me along like I was a ninety year old woman. I should respect his kind gesture, but I really do prefer to walk to the bathroom alone. He even waited for me outside the door! Then he guided me back to my chair. Leading me out onto the dance floor, he was so close that he stepped on my heal, breaking my shoe strap. While we danced, he tightly secured his arms around me as if we had been lovers for years. Later we went out for a bite to eat and I changed his name to "the spitter." When he spoke, he sprayed me with little dabs of spit. During dinner, I took cover behind the flowered centerpiece. All evening I tried to nonchalantly wipe spit off my face. Oh, the poor man. Double Oh, poor me! Sometimes I wonder if I'm being too picky with men. Maybe I need to get down off this pedestal.

September 13, 1992

On est arriveé a PARIS! I've made it to Paris! I'm really here in France with Sheila and Marlene! We've already spent ten days being the ultimate tourists in this fabulous city of stone! Our hotel room is small and there are no screens on the windows, but I guess there are no mosquitoes here. I don't particularly like the bidet in the bathroom nor the fact that there is not a real shower nozzle or curtain. Instead, there is a long hose attached to the faucet. And it's got a life of its own. The three of us have our own method of shampooing: I squeeze the hose between my knees; Sheila puts it underneath her leg; and Marlene turns the water on at the very last possible minute. Any way you do it, the bathroom gets soaked! I can't use my blow dryer because the plugs are different. Other than that, Paris is wonderful! So far: we've walked through *Palais de Chaillot*, *Champ de Mars*, and saw the Eiffel Tower! The ascent up that huge and majestic monument of steal is amazing!

Took a cab down to the *Arc de Triomphe*. That was a frightful white knuckle ride. Climbed the top of the *Arc*, and later decided to walk down *Champs-Elysées*. We had had enough driving on the

Impossible Choices

wrong side of the road. Marlene was appalled that she had to pay 2 francs to use a public bathroom. We have visited the sensational art museum, the *Lourve*. It is impossible to see every exhibit in one day.

What an international nightmare day! The three of us split up because Marlene wanted to spend a few hours visiting her old neighborhood where she had been a Nanny. Sheila decided to take a bus to *Pigalle* which is the equivalent to the Combat Zone in Boston. She wanted to buy a sexy negligee and French perfume at one of those shops. I don't have a man to go home to and showoff such things, so I made a brainless decision to venture out on my own in a foreign city. What in the world was I thinking?! I took four years of Spanish in high school! What was I doing in France? Although I have always been told that French and Spanish are similar... they're not similar enough. Sheila took French in school, but after hearing Marlene dispute Sheila's phrases and correct every little thing she says, I'm not so sure Sheila faired any better than me today!

So I dared to take the Metro which is ten times bigger than our subway system! Of course I became extremely lost immediately. If I didn't look like the saddest tourist wearing my fanny pack snug around my waist, my camera hanging off my shoulder, and a dumb expression across my face! Asked a guard—with a killer dog who never stopped yapping at me—at the station of *Montparnasse* how to get to *Musée Marmottan*. Marlene had written a few notes, but they didn't seem to help. I just kept babbling in English to anyone who would listen.

Finally, I got to my destination... where I got thrown out for taking a picture of the parquet floor! I could see if I was snapping shots of the art on the walls. On the way back to our hotel, I was delirious with fatigue, and not in the mood for the fellow passen-

Barbara Dooling

gers! For one thing, the seating is so close together, your knees touch the other person! As usual, I had to go to the bathroom, only I now had to go number two. I felt an attack of diarrhea coming on! I think the raw steak and stinky *fromage* (cheese) I ate last night at *Place de l'Alma* made me sick. Not that I didn't try to send the meat back by asking the waiter, "Por favor!" I don't think the meal was bad, just different. I'm not used to these rich creamy sauces and cuisine of multi cheeses! So this is gourmet?! Better stick to my usual "estrogen" chicken! So searching for toilettes became a part of my crazy day.

Back on the train, it was traveling so fast, I thought I was in the death seat. A guy across from me was rubbing a stain from his crotch. The one on my right smelled so gross of body odor and he kept rubbing his legs against mine. Two woman on my left were carrying on a conversation in some unknown language (not French). Miss Japan was two seats over, sitting quietly, but aggressively picking her nose… and me? I was wondering where all the Parisian people were. Getting off that train, I tried to talk to a man whom I thought was French. What a mistake! He had bad breath and the most awful teeth. Such a crummy ending to a long day! I couldn't wait to get back to the room to make this entry!

Sheila and Marlene had a much better experience! Sheila finally found her you know what at *Pigalle* and also bought Coco perfume! She had wine at a quaint outdoor café with *chevre* (goat cheese), French onion soup, and cauliflower and broccoli pate. Marlene came back with Paco Rabanne perfume, a Christian Dior purse for $400 (God only knows how many francs that is), saw a few street entertainers… a dwarf with big hands, a juggler, and a unitard with a whistle. She had *crepes* for lunch with two cups of coffee—first espresso, then café au lait. I was lucky to come back

Impossible Choices

with my few postcards which took me nearly an hour to buy because I was clueless on the money exchange! I bought a bottle of water for lunch with 22 francs and figured out later that was five dollars! Can you imagine! Just the same, I was quite proud of my adventure!

Went to *La Tour Maine Montparnasse* to the top floor for drinks. What a spectacular view of Paris! Sheila ordered one bottle of *Moet et Chandon* champagne for 390 francs, Marlene and I each ordered a glass of wine. After the wine, I bought a glass of champagne from Sheila! Hah, Hah! While we were sipping Moet, the lights on the *Eiffel Tower* and the *Arc de Triomphe* all went out at exactly 1:00 AM. It seemed as though the lights in the whole city went off. The following day we enjoyed a boat ride on *Bateau Mouche* along the *River Seine*.

Another day was spent at *Epernay*, touring Moet & Chandon wine cellars. There were lots of dust bunnies hanging from the ceilings and on top of all the bottles, (make that elephant bunnies). We each bought a bottle of champagne, and those bottles got so heavy to carry that we eventually popped them open right inside a park filled with people. We drank them and that solved that problem quickly enough!

One of the most interesting things we've done so far, was taking a train to see the chateaus out in the country. They are breathtaking! *Versailles* is stunning! There is so much history here! The parks are lined with gardens full of beautiful flowers. I've been wishing that I was here with the man of my dreams.

Nonetheless, I am having a ball. Our American cuisine doesn't compare to the main courses with rich sauces, and the mouthwatering deserts, French pastry, and heavenly chocolates. They do indeed serve French fries in France, only with vinegar. Sheila tried to return her wine because she said it was terrible and it tasted like vinegar. The waiter politely told her that what she had poured in her glass was vinegar!

Despite our fatigue from all this site-seeing, we went to the midnight show at the Lido. We were in line on the *Champs-Elysées* with half of Spain! Now this was okay with me! Except one lady tried to cut in front of us, and I spoke right up and said, "*Pardon, Madame,*" and bodily removed her by gently putting my hands on her shoulders and escorting her behind us. We waited in that line for a very long time, and when we finally entered the club, Sheila asked for a table for one! Ha, ha and she thinks she's so cool! The THREE of us were led to the bar, but actually ended up sitting at a table center stage. A perfect location to see feathers everywhere! The ice skaters were the best—boobs everywhere. The costumes and sets were beautiful especially the fountains, skating rink, future space, fire in a volcano, waterfall, and a cowboy set! They even had live animals on stage. I've never seen anything like it! The evening cost us 305 francs each ($65.00).

Today we had picnic in Claude Monet's garden in the quaint town of *Giverny*. We followed a path that lead to the water lily pond where many of the lilies were blooming. Entering Monet's pink house was like being in a garden filled with colorful flowers. Lots of family photos hung on the pastel colored walls. We ascended up a creaky old narrow staircase to the bedrooms; each one had its own view of the lily pond. Monet's room was painted yellow (including the armoire). Downstairs in the dining room, was a beautiful tablecloth embroidered with blue irises. The china was yellow and blue, and a fireplace displayed blue marble and blue tiles. Every room in the house was full of bright colors. It's obvious Monet loved color! We have also seen the magnificent Opera

Impossible Choices

House, which looks more like a huge castle. And speaking of castles, we walked up the many, many stairs to *Sacré Coeur*—a gorgeous white church that has a tremendous view of Paris. Tomorrow we'll visit *Notre Dame*. I have never done so much walking. The days are long and the nights—longer! What a sensational trip!

October 3, 1992

Mary had another baby today and she let me help coach in the delivery room with Eddie. It's a girl! Baby Alicia came into our world with red hair and strong lungs! She's precious. Mary and I cried; what a beautiful experience it was to witness this new life! They've asked me to be Alicia's godmother. I'm already godmother to their son Christopher. I'm touched and honored. Of course I said yes. Now Mom and Dad have thirteen grandchildren! What an unbelievable change in them over these past few years. I am just so proud. It gives me special joy to see Mom and Dad "living" happily! The grandchildren give them eternal smiles and bring them laughter and brighter days than I think they've ever known. God, I hope they live to see my children. They must!

October 24, 1992

Tonight of all nights—a Halloween party—I finally met the real Santa Claus. Mary, Sheila, and I donned costumes and went; we hadn't planned on going since Mary just had the baby two weeks ago. But Sheila and I persuaded her to leave Alicia home with her brother and daddy. I conjured up a costume from an old black lace party dress. I wore black lace nylon stockings and bought some gaudy black and gold jewelry. I crowned my head with a colorful Spanish Tiara that I made out of a long black scarf with bright red roses. I pinned a red rose at my cleavage and wore red high heal

Barbara Dooling

sandals. My hands were covered with black lace gloves, and I made a fancy thirty-one year old Senorita if I say so myself! I believe Santa spotted me right away—just as soon as we walked in the door. All three of us were staring into the crowded room in order to find a place to sit. We were late and there were only two seats left at a table with Santa. I didn't want to sit there because Santa had brought two friends dressed as huge Christmas gifts. I thought the boxes would block my view of the dance floor. Since we had no choice, we plunked down next to Santa. Out of the corner of my eye, I could see him stealing glances at me. I secretly watched him, too. Mary and Sheila kept nudging me to ask him to dance. They were inconspicuously scooting me over toward Santa inch-by-inch. Whenever they came back from the bar or the little girls room, they would shuffle the chairs a bit closer.

All evening, girls paraded over, joking and sitting on his lap asking plenty for Christmas. Their lists were long. In quick revolving shifts, one-by-one, they asked for a yacht, a Porsche, and still another wanted a diamond and a Harley Davidson. Dear old St. Nick finally mustered up the nerve to ask me what I wanted for Christmas. I didn't sit on his lap like those teasing ladies... I foolishly answered; "a kitty." I guess Santa figured he could come through with the cat so he asked me to dance. We danced the night away.

He liked my answer, and I guess he was quite fancied with my black lacy dress, too. As for me, I was captured by his spirited and warm smile underneath that heavy white beard. Santa and the Spanish Senorita danced to *Love Shack* by the B 52's. If we didn't look totally opposite! But it was a blast! In that red suit, Santa appeared to be cute. He is short... like me (drats, but after a few songs, I barely noticed). Santa was very soft spoken and all I could

Impossible Choices

see of him behind those bushy white eyebrows was his beautiful green eyes. Those eyes were as docile as his voice. Although he introduced me to his friends Joe and Cindy, I don't think either of us spoke to our companions the rest of the evening. Nope, except for a few polite words, and general small talk with first-time acquaintance type questions, Santa and I seemed to be in our own world.

I kept wondering what he looked like beneath that costume! I couldn't tell if he was bald, or his hair was gray, or punk orange! The beard covered most of his face except for those dreamy eyes and his flawless cheeks. No wrinkles, blemishes, or scars, I'm guessing that he's about twenty-seven, maybe twenty-eight. Likewise, he couldn't see my hair! I was so hot from dancing, yet I didn't dare take my tiara off. I was praying it would stay on top of my head through all the bouncing. Underneath, I knew it was matted down and drenched with sweat. We danced so much that I had to pat my forehead and neck with a cocktail napkin to remove the beads of perspiration. The Senorita was wilting like a bouquet of Valentine roses left near a radiator. Like those drooping buds, one-by-one, things started to fall apart on me. My makeup was running, and the mascara melted on top and below my eyelids. I was beginning to look like a real mess. Luckily he couldn't see the dribbles that rolled down between my breasts. I don't have much cleavage but that dress is skin tight and gives my boobs a lift. Gee, he said I'm a good dancer. When we slow danced, the pillow he'd stuffed under the red jacket kept our bodies from fitting together. That was kind of funny, but I rested against him just the same, and he smelled like *Obsession eau de toilette*. I think it's a men's cologne by Calvin Klein. At least he had an enticing scent… I'm not sure what the heck I smelled like! Having four brothers, I know my scents.

81

Barbara Dooling

Back at the table, I turned to Mary and Sheila who were trying to talk over the loud music, and casually told them to "beat it, get lost, disappear!" I smiled nonchalantly, motioned my eyes in the direction of the crowd at the bar and repeated, "Get lost!"

They did! As for Joe and Cindy, Tom must have given them the boot too; they stayed out on the dance floor the rest of the night. By this time, it was nearly midnight and I just knew I'd turn into a pumpkin when the hall lights were flipped on during last call for drinks. Santa finagled his drenched body out of that suit, and I was praying he didn't suggest I remove the tiara. He wore faded jeans with a black T shirt, and black cowboy boots. His hair is brown! And he has lots of it! Well, I was keeping that tiara fixed on my head if I had to hold it in place! No way could I let him see my hair askew! Before the evening was over, Santa (his name's really Tom) had Senorita's phone number.

October 26, 1992

It's been three solid days and Santa hasn't called yet. Not to push the panic button until Saturday. Guys usually call (if they're going to call) by Friday to go out over the weekend. It's only Tuesday. I hate waiting for men to call me. I loathe being a prisoner to the phone… each time it rings, I kill myself to reach the receiver, then answer casually as though I was home dusting the furniture. It's not like me to be a P.O.W., prisoner of "waiting," prisoner of "wishing," prisoner of "wistful"! I'm more like fancy free, carefree, freewheeling, freethinker! Oh, but why doesn't that darn phone ring?! Stay calm, Barbara. Keep busy. Hey, if he doesn't call… no big deal. Come to think of it, he's kind of short. In fact, if I wore high heels, I'd be taller than him!

Impossible Choices

October 27, 1992
 No call. No Call. NO CALL!

October 28, 1992
 If one more telemarketer calls this house! If the Boston Globe thinks I want to subscribe! If a single charity requests a contribution! If an exceptional company solicits their superior product that I supposedly can't and shouldn't be living without! If a solitary individual inquires about some vital survey! I'm going to scrrrreeeaaam! What is with these people? Get a life, get a real job! Get off the phone! Get off my phone!

October 29, 1992
 Hello, Santa! Howz the weather up at the North Pole? What's Rudolph been up to? Has Herby got his D.M.D. yet? Is he keeping your teeth pearly white? How are the other elves faring with making all the toys? Just fifty-six more days till Christmas, you know. Tell them to get busy. And Mrs. Clause? What's that you say? There is no Mrs.? Well, I'd be happy to take a sleigh ride with you! I'd be delighted to soar past the clouds, and venture to your cabin. Yes, I do have a parka and I'll be sure to bring my quilt.

 I'm ecstatic! Mr. Kringle and I have made plans for dinner and to see the play *Forever Plaid*. Tom was able to get tickets for tomorrow night's performance. Hopefully we won't be watching from up in the rafters! No matter, I'm just psyched he called! He can't be all that short.

October 31, 1992
 Our date last night was quite pleasant!!!!!! There were no fireworks, bells or whistles, but there is something about this guy that

comforts me. He's just so nice. We both seemed relaxed and there was no putting on airs.

Our night began at the Purity Supreme parking lot rather than my house. He knows exactly where the supermarket is, so we figured that might be easier. I was dressed a bit formal for buying bread and milk, although I'm sure people swing into the market after work. There I waited, looking rather chic in my ebony suede skirt with black silk stockings, my hunter green silk blouse, a gold jacquard blazer ornately decorated with green and copper leaves, accented with a wide chamois green belt with gold buckle that rested snugly around my thin waistline. It was a bit odd to just be hanging out, leaning against my car, scanning the lot for Santa Claus.

Luckily, he pulled up precisely at six. We were both punctual, and he had a lovely bouquet of autumn flowers. After we exchanged hellos and I gave him a peck on the cheek, we got back into our separate cars, circled around the block, and he followed me to the apartment so I could drop off my car. I invited him in for a cold drink while I put the orange tiger lilies, yellow and gold mums, and a splash of baby's breath in a vase. Bruce was vegging on the couch, catching the news and weather. I introduced the two men and wondered if Tom would try to draw any conclusions about the living arrangements. Other men I've dated have done this. Some were quite jealous of my relationship with Bruce even though we are just friends. Bruce tried his best to strike up a casual conversation with Tom. The flowers were in water so it was time to go. Tom took the lead out, and as I closed the front door behind us, I winked at Bruce, and Bruce whispered and laughed at the same time, "He seems nice. Don't screw this up. I don't plan to live with you forever, you know."

We ate at Legal Seafood's in the heart of the theater district. Our

Impossible Choices

meals of swordfish and baked stuffed lobster were scrumptious. The vegetables and salad were savory with mild spices. The musical was hilarious. It was a bit more geared for people who grew up in the 1950's and early 60's, but we really enjoyed it. After the show, Tom curled my arm into his and we strolled along the noisy streets until we settled at Jacob Worth's pub for a nightcap. I feel like I did most of the talking... he's a bit quiet without the support of loud music and people in costume occasionally interacting. Bruce claims that the poor guy probably couldn't get a word in edgewise with the way I ramble on. Hate to admit it, but he might be right!

Oops, be right back, have to pass out some Halloween candy to some trick-or-treaters. How adorable they look! We haven't had many kids. I know it's because Bruce lined the walkway with sixteen pumpkins, eight on each side, carved into the most scary jack-o'-lanterns. The children are literally frightened to come up to the steps. The sculptures do look cool with their chiseled fangs and very large circled eyes! This is an annual ritual for Bruce, and he always does a super job! Unfortunately, the little ones don't appreciate his artistic expression! Bruce just loves to scare the pants off the kids, and he watches intently out the window to see them scurry past the house. The mommies and daddies attempt to walk toward our path, but the children yank on their arms and drag their parents away! It is pretty funny! We won't be laughing if our house gets egged.

I wore my Spanish outfit, and each time I answered the door, I danced in circles clicking and clapping castanets above my head. The kids had no clue what I was, and the parents probably thought I was too old for such silliness, but I love Halloween!

So my date with Santa Claus ended with another innocent smooch... not on the lips. But he cupped my face in both of his

Barbara Dooling

hands and planted that kiss right on my forehead. His hands were firm yet delicate, and his lips were moist and left a tingling sensation for a long moment. Our good-bye was simple and quick. He asked me out again already... no waiting for his call! He wants to get together during the week, but I told him with my work schedule, sometimes I don't get home until after seven, and I'm wiped out. Then he mentioned this coming Friday night, except that I had planned on visiting my grandmother in the nursing home. I explained to Tom that my Nana was just placed in the convalescent home only a few weeks ago. She's ninety-three years old, and has been lucky enough to live on her own all this time. Now she is failing a bit—forgetting to take her medicine or taking it incorrectly, starting fires in the kitchen when she's cooking, and falling in the bathroom. I hate to see Nana lose her independence, but the circumstances warrant this change.

I couldn't believe it when Tom asked if he could join me on my visit to Nana's. Sure thing, if he considers it a fun date sitting in a steaming hot lounge with gray-haired folks slumped in wheelchairs, screaming obscenities or calling out to people who died long ago to come get them out of the place. That's what it's like all right, and if you can get past the smell, tune out the wacky shouting, steady your feet flat on the floor when someone shrieks and scares the heck out of ya, and stop yourself from crying, it might not be so bad. I truly loathe the place. However, I've seen ancient souls there like Nana who have most of their faculties, and can surely tell a good story.

November 7, 1992

Our second date couldn't have been nicer, although Nana kept calling Tom, Bruce. Well, at least she has the right person with the

Impossible Choices

correct association. Tom was an absolute doll! He charmed Nana and all the rest of the folks who were up late enough to see us. He kept fixing a blanket, or helping with a sweater, and pouring little cups of water for everyone. Nana would say, "Thank you, Bruce." I'd remind her of his real name, but she kept it up all night. Eventually, Tom said to let her be. I plunked away on the piano, striking the keys clumsily because all I know how to play is *Twinkle, Twinkle Little Star* and *Mary Had a Little Lamb*. But the residents thought I was a regular at the night club they used to frequent or Liberace himself! On the way out back to the parking garage, Tom stole a kiss in the elevator. Still just a tap on the cheek. It's my own doing, I keep offering the side of my face rather than my lips. I'm such a prude! I hope he doesn't think I'm a tease. I just don't like getting mauled by someone I hardly know.

November 11, 1992

Today is Veterans Day and neither Tom nor I had the day off, but we managed to play hooky. We were good little patriots and enjoyed a pizza together at a joint near his apartment in Arlington. Tom is renting the top floor of a two family home that his mom and her four siblings grew up in. He showed me around but we didn't stay too long. It has lots of antiques: furniture, dishes, vases, and all sorts of stuff that had belonged to his grandmother. He was very close to "Grammy" and says he feels her presence in the house. He visited her grave and told her about me! It seems like this guy is very sensitive… AND sentimental! Anyway, our afternoon was cut short, because I really had to get home and work on some reports that I took home, knowing that I was going to call in a mental health day. He got the tongue! But just one kiss.

Barbara Dooling

November 14, 1992

I fell in love with Santa last night. Could this be it? Could I have met my prince charming? My night in shining armor invited me to his apartment for dinner. Our fourth Date!!!! With trepidation, I accepted his invitation, wondering what no-good he was up to. Boy, did I ever get the shock of my life... Tom rented "G" rated *Beauty and The Beast* and cooked for dinner a delectable feast, complete with chilled Champaign! These were his wicked intentions. We talked until four in the morning and that was it. Okay, honestly? He got far more than the cheek this time but we didn't sleep together. Never did "IT." Our conversation was comfortable and free from nervous small talk. We were so relaxed together rattling away without pause about our families, our jobs, and our dreams. I was not afraid to scare him off with talk about wishing for a great guy and children. Tom revealed that he wants the same thing. He also dreams about owning a Harley Davidson. I'm not sure which order he wants these things.

When Tom kissed me last night, I felt like I had been woken out of a deep sleep. My heart was fluttering like a frightened rabbit. Might he be the one to break the spell? He is amazingly kind and gentle. His kisses were slow and sensuous, and not limited to my lips. In the slightest way, he allowed his tongue to tenderly stroke my neck. I felt my blood rushing to my face. I'm sure my cheeks were flush. His tongue continued to stray back to my lips, parting them until it was inside my mouth. He fingered my hair, taming the little snarls that matted during those hours on the couch. He thinks I'm pretty! I think I love him! I know I do!

November 24, 1992

I cooked him an Italian dinner at my place. I had to get rid of

Impossible Choices

Bruce for the evening, but Bruce was good about it. As the scrumptious aroma of spaghetti sauce and chicken cutlets filled the apartment, Bruce said, "I'll just make myself a peanut butter and jelly sandwich and go sit out on the curbside for the night. You have a great time and don't bother about me!" After Bruce left with his sarcasm, I set a lovely table with candles and wine. Being like my mother, I had antipasto, salad, and all kinds of Italian appetizers like artichoke hearts, peppers, brochette and several types of cheese. How could I have forgotten that my new boyfriend(?) was Irish? The poor guy was turning green trying to be polite and eat everything. Basically the only thing he liked was the chicken. I would have been better off with a boiled dinner! Ugh! Half of the appetizers wound up in his napkin and the antipasto was anti-eaten... he never touched it or his salad. He kindly said that everything was wonderful, especially the artichoke hearts, and we both roared with laughter.

December 19, 1992

Tom and I went to the Nutcracker at The Wang Center in Boston with Joe and Cindy. I was in my glory with good seats and a stunning performance by the Boston Ballet. The guys did not appreciate the show, but I think Cindy liked it. I loved it!

We all went out for cocktails after the matinee. Joe and Tom have been best friends since they were ten years old—almost as long as Sheila and I. They are like brothers. Joe is an only child, and although Tom has four siblings, they are all girls. We shared a lot of laughs while Joe filled me in on some crazy stories about their youth. Tom and Joe never kissed posters, but they wore platform shoes, polyester shirts, and Aqua-Velva after shave to the junior high school dances despite the fact that neither of them shaved. Joe claims that he and Tom were cool dudes, but Tom admitted to being a wallflower. They have traded in their platforms for biker boots and leisure suits for black leather jackets. Joe already owns a Harley, and Tom rides a Honda. He plans on trading up someday. Cindy claims to enjoy a free ride through back country roads. I'd be white knuckled, clinging for life, and silently praying. Surely I'd cause a spill fighting to tilt in the opposite direction instead of leaning into a turn. I'd embarrass Tom with my pastel clothing! Well, I do have a suede jacket, but it's bronze, not black. Cindy's got the whole kit and caboodle: riding coat, chaps, helmet. And she's tall, slender, and blond—she's gorgeous. She only dresses in all that leather when they go riding.

After a couple of drinks following the show, the four of us went to Tom's sister Tricia's house where there was a small family gathering for his niece Devan's birthday. Yep, I met the whole "famdamily" all at once! At least I was dressed to the 9s. Everyone was really nice. Tom appears to be close to all of his four sisters and the brother-in-laws to boot. There was so much chatter and laughter. It's the "big family" syndrome. I just love it!

Tricia and I hit it off immediately. She has two Claude Monet prints hanging in the living room, and the house is dazzled with Victorian décor. What lovely taste. She's five months pregnant with her third child, and still full of energy being the perfect hostess. Margaret who is the oldest, has three children. She's quite congenial, cheerful and when she laughs her entire face blushes. She calls Tom: Thomas. So do his parents. I told his mom Alice that she raised a perfect gentleman. She ate it right up. But I wasn't trying to impress her; it's the truth! Big Tom is Tom's dad. And, he is big. He's got thick, wavy, silver hair—more hair than me! I really like Big Tom, he's soft spoken, except when he's shouting at the grandchildren

Impossible Choices

who are running through the house, causing quite a ruckus. Every now and again, his dad referred to me as, "Young Lady." He would ask, "And what do you do for work, Young Lady?" Or he'd say, "So Young Lady, tell me about your folks." Big Tom is just a love! I'm sure Tom gets his tender voice from his dad. Alice is a howl. She is very high-spirited and full of wisecracks that keep everyone in hysterics. Hmm... so his wit comes from his mom. Carolyn and Donna are the two younger sisters. Carolyn seems honest and plainspoken, very frank. Donna is a doll! She's petite like me, has gorgeous long blond hair, and the most beautiful blue eyes I've ever seen. She's outgoing and loads of fun. I like this family. I hope they like me.

December 20, 1992

Payback is a B—CH! Mary and Eddie had a Christmas brunch. Now it was Tom's turn to meet my gang. What I love about Tom is that he doesn't try to impress anyone, yet he impresses by just being his sincere ol' self. He made himself right at home, helping Mary make coffee, and clear the table. This is not for show. He does it all the time at my apartment and at his own. Mom and Dad seem to be quite fond of him. This is a crash "Dating and Family Dynamics" course for both of us. Between the holiday gatherings and all this socializing, things are happening very fast! Our relationship is taking off like a jet.

December 24, 1992

Our first Christmas! We had a tree decorating party with Champagne, strawberries, and chocolates. Yummy! Something about that bubbly stuff that gets me going if you know what I mean. Seems to me they go hand and hand: sparkling wine and lovin. There was no stopping him tonight; he took me right there beneath

Barbara Dooling

the partially decorated tree. It's all his fault. While I was innocently trying to get some bulbs on his tree, he pinched my toosh. I whipped around to slap his hand and before I could catch my balance he grabbed for a boob! I told him he was being naughty, and he scooped me in his arms and kissed me for a long time. He gently lowered us both to the floor, and slowly began to undress me. I let him. Limp with satisfaction, I gazed up at the tiny lights, and the glittering garland. This time, I followed his lead, unlike when we are dancing. Our lovemaking made its way into the bedroom where there was nothing shy about this man. He took his time, and caressed every inch of my body like no other man has ever done. When we were finished loving each other, he held me tightly under the grip of his shoulder, turned my chin with his hand to face me toward his expression, and he said, "I love you Barbara Goyette." His eyes were filled with truth; he squeezed me as if to put an exclamation after that "I love you." I told him that I wanted to spend the rest of my life with him, and he replied, "An eternity!"

January 1, 1993

Rang in the new year together—over and over and over again! He is relentless in bed! Slow, steady, and sensuous! He takes great steps to satisfy me. He's incredibly in-tuned with what pleases a woman! We did not stray far from the house today. For that matter, we hardly left the bedroom except to sneak to the bathroom or have a quick bite to eat.

January 16, 1993

Every weekend and some weeknights, Tom either stays at my apartment or we stay at his. I just knew we'd get caught one of these days. At thirty-two, I still feel like a kid when it comes to our

Impossible Choices

parents. And so on this sixteenth day in January, when his mom dropped by his apartment, there I was with guilt plastered all over my flushed face. Oh the fact that I was there on a Saturday morning wasn't so bad... it was my luggage and clothing so comfortably strewn about the place. Topping it off, Alice was with Tom's Uncle Howard who is a man of the cloth! I was embarrassed and Tom was shaking with stifled laughter. I could see it in his eyes. He whispered, "Shall I invite them to stay for tea and ask them to help make the bed?" What a brat. I told him I'd take care of him later, but he only said that he couldn't wait.

January 30, 1993

I'm sneaking a passage in my precious journal before I must join Tom and his sisters by a blazing fire in the wood stove. I am scribbling with haste. We've all had a full day of skiing and now we are resting comfortably in his parents' cozy cottage in Maine. It is my first time away with Carolyn and Donna. I think they do like me—hope so. Everyone is exhausted, which is typical after getting up before dawn and spending a day working out on the slopes. Tom spent the entire day with me on the intermediate hills because I'm just a mediocre skier. I thought it was so nice of him to give up the excitement of moguls and steeper, more challenging terrain. But we laughed all day at my clumsy style, and he taught me some new helpful positions. He stole a kiss on my numb lips right there on the top of Mount Sunday River. The view was awesome. We both stood speechless for a moment while we admired the snow covered mountains. The sun was blinding as it reflected off the stark white snow. My eyes were tearing up and I was unsure if it was the wonder of that moment or the strong sun.

Barbara Dooling

February 6, 1993

Sunning myself on a Cancun beach with Tom! The slight breeze is cooling to my hot skin. The blazing sun is scorching! Back home it is a cold raw New England winter with the inevitable chance of snow, and here we sit with beads of perspiration trickling on our face and body. I wonder what the poor folks in frigid Boston are doing? Tee hee hee!

I always carry bubbles in my beach bag, and I just made new friends with some local children. I tried to remember Spanish from my high school days, but my memory failed me. I came up with very few words, but we sure had plenty of laughs as the Chicos chased the bubbles all over that beach. The wind took those shiny delicate, glistening balls floating right into the air—each displaying a rainbow until it popped. After playing, I gave my bottle of fun to the little ones. Tom and I tread water in the sensational warm green sea, and talked of our future together. It is truly grand that he loves the ocean, too. We like a lot of the same things. He says we're two peas in a pod. I am loving this day... this moment with him. He reaches across the blanket and takes my journal and pen away from me. He curls his strong hand around my small fingers, and leans into me for a soft kiss on the lips. We lay together until we both slip into a comfortable doze. The sun warms our bodies. I am so content with this man.

February 13, 1993

Tom took me to see *Beauty and the Beast on Ice*, a Disney performance at the Boston Garden arena. The place was filled with children and their parents, but it was a fine date for us! I was thrilled to see the show! How sweet of Tom to think of getting these tickets. He is such a sensitive man and he knows just what

Impossible Choices

makes me smile. Tom promised that someday we would take our children to see a show. My heart was fluttering with extra beats. I was certain if it weren't for all the noise, he would have heard it pounding. He turns 30 in ten days; I want to do something special. I don't know how I will top this wonderful evening, but I shall try. I might kidnap him and steal away to some fancy hotel.

February 19, 1993

Tonight I gathered twenty of our closest friends and family for Chinese food and a comedy show to celebrate Tom's thirtieth. His sisters and their spouses were there and most of my family was, too. It was the first time we've gotten the two clans together. A good time was had by all!

April 16, 1993

Tom bought tickets for my thirty-second birthday to see Elton John in concert tonight. It was a fabulous concert! I am truly having the time of my life!

May 15, 1993

Another wonderful evening with my love. This courtship is getting serious with lots of talk about marriage, kids, houses, dogs, cats, and his Harley. I wonder about one lady in particular that he spoke to the night we met… remember the one who told Santa she wanted a Harley for Christmas? I remember. I'm far from a Harley chick,, but I've nothing to worry about. He can have his motorcycle and I'll have my ballet. Nothing wrong with having different interests as long as you give each other space, and have common ground. We have so many other things in common: we both love the beach; we like to ski; we enjoy the great outdoors, yet we're both

Barbara Dooling

homebodies when it comes to renting a movie and sipping tea on a cold and lazy Sunday afternoon. But now the spring is here, offering many activities on sunshiny days.

June 9, 1993

This evening we took in a play with Tom's parents—*My Fair Lady*. It was lovely. Should I say that his parents really like me? Honest, I think they do!

July 12, 1993

He is constantly bringing me flowers—usually roses. I have never seen such beautiful colors: lavender, peach, and white. The purple roses have a delicious strong scent. He hasn't just flattered me with bouquets, he is forever leaving me little love notes tucked away in the medicine chest or a kitchen cabinet. Seems every time I open something, his kindness is there. One day Bruce found a message taped underneath the washing machine lid and he teased, "Here Juliet, I think this is for you from Romeo."

August 7, 1993

Tom and I have large families with lots of nieces and nephews. He is a true family-man and it shows. He is very helpful to his parents and he visits them often. Sometimes we sit for hours sipping coffee and tea enjoying pleasant conversation. His mom and dad are fine people. Their company is delightful. Between his family and mine, we are always attending a holiday gathering or someone's birthday celebration. Alice had me over for a nice Italian feast and was quite proud of her meatballs and lasagna. I was teased by Tom's sisters because she gave me a fine bone china cup and everyone else had the old chipped mugs. Likewise, my mom cooked Tom a

Impossible Choices

bloody roast beef with steamy mashed potatoes and buttery carrots. It is so funny how everyone is trying to roll out the red carpet. I knew my dad liked Tom when he gave up the one sharp knife in the house for Tom's place setting. Dad had actually marked the knife with red nail polish in order to guarantee that he'd get the right knife. And there it was, at the opposite head of the table waiting for Tom. I lifted the infamous blade and held it up to Mom. She laughed outloud.

The nieces and nephews are equally as generous to Tom and I, sharing their special toys and making colorful pictures for us to take home. Tom is wonderful with children, and I love to watch him in action. He is devoted to his sisters' little ones and now he dotes over my rug rats, too. The kids are predicting a wedding. We shall see!

September 26, 1993

Well, there's going to be a wedding all right, but not mine. Today was the bridal shower. Sheila is getting married and she's asked me to be her maid of honor. She is an only child and she told me I'm really like a sister to her. We are indeed like family... We've been friends now for twenty-seven years. We are both professionals. She's a human resource manager of a large company in Boston. Me, I'm still office manager/ fill-in medical assistant/do-everything girl for the Internal Medicine doctors. So Sheila is departing the single scene and I'm so happy for her. Good-bye Donny Osmond, no more kissing Robert Wagner. Sheila will have a real living breathing husband of her very own. Ha, Ha!

It's going to be such fun picking out her wedding gown and helping Sheila plan the grand affair. Mary, Marlene, and Julie will be in the wedding, too. What a blast we'll have! Always a maid, never a bride! This is getting to be a habit. I was maid of honor for Mary, now Sheila. And I've been a bride's maid for Geno and Karen, Paul and Maureen, my friend Denise, and for Kenny's wedding in Newport. No kidding, I've been in all those weddings! I have more gowns than one might see at the Astor's grand ball. At least I've had a few occasions to wear them again... Marlene always hosts a black-tie party on the evening of the Academy Awards. We have our own ceremony with real trophies and speeches. It is hysterical! While we watch it aired on TV, the guys strut and showoff in tuxedos, top hats, and tails with walking sticks. The woman wear old prom or bridesmaids' gowns, long white gloves, and hold unlit cigarettes attached to a long black stick. It's the greatest time!

October 23, 1993

Today was the day!!! So unbelievable was this day that I was actually in denial that it is all happening to me. I'm thirty-two and my dream has come true! It can't be real, I must be fantasizing again. Surely this is just another fairy tale daydream...

But wait... it is truly my life. I know this is real because I'm still trembling as I write this. I have a few moments to sneak an entry. Tom has gone to get ice for drinks and wood for a fire. We're at the lovely Trapp Family Lodge in Stowe, Vermont. This was originally the home of the Von Trapp family from the movie, *The Sound of Music*. One of my favorite classics! It's such a romantic place to spend the weekend! The most amazing thing—and surely this is proof that we are soulmates—was that we gave each other the same anniversary card. How revealing is that? The exact same card! And we both secretly brought *Beauty and the Beast* trinkets along to decorate the room. How astonishing! I brought the storybook and two little figurines of Belle and Beast. I snuggled them together on the night

Impossible Choices

stand as soon as we arrived. The next thing I knew, a silly plastic flashlight, holding the enchanted rose, was resting with Belle and Beast. Tom had borrowed this Disney toy from his little niece Devan. How silly two adults are smuggling toys and children's books into a hotel for decorations. Lovers are of course the silliest people.

Among all our *Beauty and the Beast* Treasures, Tom placed red and yellow roses. The message on the little card read: "yellow is for friendship and red is for love. I'm glad I found both in you." Oh how sweet, isn't he the sweetest man? Don't ask me how he managed to sneak the roses and keep them from wilting during the five hour drive to Vermont. See? I knew God had a noble prince for me who would make all my dreams come true.

This is the last day of the weekend and prince charming saved a grand finalé of a surprise. You have to admit, he really is a prince. I was actually more surprised than you might imagine since we'd never gone looking for engagement rings. On our first evening in this romantic lodge, he threw me off by giving me a pair of gold earrings as an anniversary present. They were indeed very lovely and I was quite happy. I did not imagine there was anything else.

But today... we were out walking through a very old and unique cemetery at the edge of the lodge's sprawling grounds, and he nervously pulled the ring out of his pocket. Right in the middle of the cemetery! I had no idea what he was doing. I just stood there astonished as he asked me to be his wife. Tom said we would begin our lives together there, until death do us part. My knees felt like water; they no longer wanted to support my shaking body. I threw my arms around him and burst into tears. I just couldn't believe this was happening to me. The unmarried aunt is getting married next autumn!

Barbara Dooling

The air was so cold and crisp. Trees were painted with striking colors. Some had already lost their foliage. Lots of bright splashes covered the ground. The brown leaves were rustling and crunching beneath our feet. As we walked arm and arm, we kicked at the dry leaves. Then, very peacefully, snow flurries began to float down around us—a perfect day! My heart has been captured. The afternoon sun quickly set, nudging the autumn moon to awaken to its full glory. It was huge and so low on the horizon one might have been able to throw a lasso and pluck it right out of the sky. We held each other so tightly and kissed the longest kiss.

Tonight we sipped Champaign by a roaring fire in our private living room. Tom kept adding more wood. The flames flickered and the wood crackled until it was so hot my face was flush, (although perhaps it was his kisses or the Champaign that roused me). I kept staring at the sparkling pear-shaped diamond with two smaller pear stones on either side. Stunning! I've never owned anything as beautiful. At that moment, Tom said, "Beautiful," but he was looking right into my eyes and not at the diamond. Calls home followed as I cried—not quite composed—There'll be a royal wedding soon, Prince Charming has proposed!

October 24, 1993

My dreams are coming true before my very eyes. Today as we drove home from our memorable weekend, Tom told me all about the way he asked my parents for their consent to marry me. He did it without my knowledge. Being very old-fashioned, my parents ate it right up! I can just see Tom now, mustering up the courage to have that "heart-to-heart" with Dad. The two men walked across the yard together and Tom revealed his love for me, asking Dad for his permission to marry his baby girl. Tom told Dad that he loved his

Impossible Choices

daughter with all his heart and he wanted to make me happy. There was a firm handshake, and they went into the house to tell Mom.

November 20, 1993

Sheila tied the knot today! She looked lovely. This time when I played the roll of maid, I did it with glee knowing that next year this time, I'll be married too! Tom kept winking at me from his spot in the pew. I could feel his warmth and love going right through my body. I fussed over straightening Sheila's train at the alter each time she moved. At the hall, my duties were not needed as much, and Tom and I became one with the dance floor. What a party! I'm really tired and my feet are killing me! Tom and I got a hotel room for this evening. He is sitting on the edge of the bed rubbing my sore toes and the balls of my feet. It's time to put the pen down...

December 25, 1993

What a surprise! Tom gave me a beautiful hope chest for Christmas. The dark cherry wood is so shiny you can see your reflection. The front is engraved with a floral design, and the actual chest stands on four short, ball and claw legs. I like that it doesn't rest on the floor. Tucked inside the cedar chest, was two pair of infant booties. Both tiny sets were fuzzy with delicate bows. There was a pink and a blue pair. I don't how Tom thinks of such surprises. I gave him a soft black leather coat, and tucked little love notes in each pocket. The jacket didn't seem to compare to his sentiments.

February 7, 1994

Got a job offer today that I couldn't refuse. More money and the chance to manage a private Ophthalmology practice in Brookline.

Barbara Dooling

He has another office in Dedham, and he's Mom's eye doctor. Mom says he's drop-dead gorgeous and she forgets all her questions the minute he walks into the examining room. I've met him, he is nice looking, happily married and soon I'll be as well! Anyway, I'm taking the job and I start the twenty-second.

April 23, 1994

I spent this whole day trying on wedding gowns! Mary and Sheila were my maids all right; they had to help me dress and undress and put all those heavy gowns back on their hangers. It was a tiring job. Now I know why so many women want to get married from the time they are little girls. The idea of dressing like a princess in a magnificent, sparkling white beaded gown with a crown of diamonds and pearls, and a flowing shear veil is simply divine! Each gown I tried on was more beautiful than the one before. I was in my glory! I just kept crying! I was so emotional as I stared at the princess in the mirror—I did feel like a princess. I did not go home with any specific choice. As gorgeous as the gowns were, not one was the right one for me.

I stopped in at Mom and Dad's house for a quick visit and I wound up rummaging through her hope chest. That was always a favorite pastime for me when I was a little girl. It's loaded with old photographs and memorabilia. I had a mission though and sure enough, Mom's wedding gown was still there. I tried it on and it fit perfectly—well, maybe a tad snug. Wow, Mom was tiny! Her gown was a champagne pale pink with long sleeves and a cathedral length scalloped train. The entire gown was a heavy satin and it still shined like new. There were no beads, sequins or pearls, but it was truly elegant!

I waltzed around the house dipping and twirling and my dear

Impossible Choices

sweet father began to cry. He scarcely got the words out, but he said, "You look stunning, Barbie." I don't suppose he had seen that dress in fifty years—that's how long Mom and Dad have been married. Fifty years with the same person? How impressive. Such commitment! As a new bride-to-be, my heart is filled with promise of all rainbows. I took mom's gown off and we all shared a hot cup of tea. The gown was indeed stunning, but I still wasn't sure it was for me. I was thinking maybe something more sparkling like Cinderella's gown.

Yesterday my birthday came and went. Tom treated me to a romantic dinner at The Hampshire House in Boston. The cake should have had thirty-three candles. Instead, Tom covered it with yellow and red roses.

May 7, 1994

I'm getting tired of house hunting every free weekend. We have tried to make the best of it by packing a lunch and stopping to picnic midday. At first it was exciting to be buying a house. After seeing homes that need so much work—more than a face lift—it was discouraging. Some of these places needed body parts and replacements! We aren't in the market for a brand new home—just can't afford it right now. We'll have to keep looking and hope the right one will appear.

June 18, 1994

"The Big Day" is right around the corner (less than 4 months) and we still haven't found a suitable home. We agreed to get an apartment, but it's going to be more difficult to save for a house. I've been packing up my things from the place Bruce and I have shared for eight years. He's like a brother. For sure I'm going to miss that guy. Not too many people can make me laugh hearty like Bruce can. I'm really glad that Tom and Bruce have become close friends. Neither of them have brothers. Tom asked Bruce to be an usher in our wedding. I'm delighted.

It was hard to decide who else will be in the wedding because we are attached to a lot of people. So we're going to have a large wedding party. Mary will be my Matron of Honor, of course. My maids and matrons will be: Sheila, Julie, Kim, Denise, and Tom's younger sister Donna. Whew! Oh yah, I must have a junior bridesmaid and a flower girl. Let's see... Tom's niece Brittany and my niece Tyla. That should do it! And the best man and ushers will be Tom's best friend Joe, his friends Mark and Bobby, his cousin Howie, my brother Geno, and Bruce. The partners for the two youngest girls will be my nephew and Godson Christopher and Tom's nephew and Godson Kevin. We'll need a fleet of limos for all these people! This is so exciting planning the wedding.

Tom's sister Tricia will do a reading. Kenny and Paul will do a reading each and together, they'll walk Mom down the aisle. I'm giving Tom a wedding poem that will be read at our reception. Russ will read the poem because I know I'll be too emotional. I'd never make it through without bawling!

August 13, 1994

Oh God, what's happening, things couldn't be worse! Dad has had a heart attack and he needs a triple bypass surgery! I just can't lose him now, God, I just can't. He has finally stopped drinking and we've had our Dad back! He has to walk me down the aisle. I've waited too long for this day. Dad has got to see me get married. I'm the last one to get married; he's got to be there! My wedding is two months away, and Mom and Dad are weeks away from celebrating

Impossible Choices

their fiftieth wedding anniversary! Mom's doing great too, she looks great, she acts great, and she is great! Oh please no, don't let Dad die! I'm terrified. I'm selfish; I want Dad to give me away—no one else. All us kids have planned a huge fiftieth party with tons of friends and relatives to attend. What's going to happen? Oh, Daddy, please don't die! I love you, Daddy; I "DO" love you, Daddy. I don't hate you, I never hated you!! Don't die Dad!

August 15, 1994

Dad survived the open heart surgery with good medical care and a lot of prayers. Not certain if he'll be well enough to walk me down the aisle, but at least he's still here. I suppose he could use a wheel chair, although, he'd never hear of that. Not my dad. I'm so grateful that we didn't lose him! I love him and Mom so much!

September 1, 1994

We've decided to get an apartment for now since we haven't had luck finding a house. Looked at a spacious flat today in Medford and put a deposit down. The owner said we could move in right away, so Tom's going to get his things in first. The place has a finished attic, two bedrooms, a large kitchen, dining room and a big living room. Wow, we'll have plenty of room for all our stuff. Nevertheless, I wish we were moving into that house in the country. You know, the one with the picket fence, dogs, cats, and kids. We want to start a family fairly soon—after all, I am thirty-three. I'd rather be settled in a house, but the apartment will have to do.

September 4, 1994

Tom and I have been making our own centerpieces for the wedding. They're just about finished. We've hand-painted twenty-four ceramic Victorian boots: ivory and burgundy with gold for the laces. Denise's mother Fran helped us fill them with burgundy roses and baby's breath. Ivory lace borders wrap the circumference of the top of the boot, and they're topped with matching burgundy velvet bows. Each guest will receive an ivory lace heart strung with burgundy ribbon and roses. With the help of Kim, Tom and I have made those too! Tom made me promise not to tell anyone that he helped with all the crafts. Night after night, we've been sitting together as we paint and string... string and paint. It's been long tedious work, but we seem to enjoy this quiet time together. He's been such a sport; I've broken my promise a hundred times telling everyone how much he's helped me!

September 7, 1994

This whole weekend we moved Tom's stuff into the apartment. Living room set, bedroom, stereo, frig, washer and dryer and all his clothes. We were pooped and sipping ice cold water on the couch when our landlord rang the door bell. He came in practically breathless and proceeded to tell us that the house had been sold! He explained that it was unexpected and he was very sorry. Tom and I just looked at each other and laughed! I said it was a good thing we hadn't moved all my things in yet. Tom called his parents who offered to let us live with them until we found another place or maybe even a house... whichever came first. Between Dad's poor health and now this, we're a bit disheveled, yet I couldn't be happier. After the landlord left us with jaws hanging, Tom lifted me off my feet and tossed me onto the couch. He settled me with gentle kisses and said we still have each other and we're getting married in a four weeks no matter what comes down around us! Yes, he's absolutely right. I love this man so much! Since my first love

Impossible Choices

back in 1979, I had doubts of finding love again. Well, I have found it.... true love... and better than before!

October 8, 1994

Our wonderful storybook wedding is tomorrow, October 9, 1994! We will marry during the harvest moon; same as the evening we met and the weekend we got engaged. The trees are blazing with color and the autumn air is comfortably cool. Pumpkins line the front stairs to Mom and Dad's house. Mom is very happy that I will be staying here tonight and getting dressed in my old room for my wedding tomorrow. The house is full of excitement and the rush of last minute things. Dad is trying on his tuxedo, Mom's making sure the house is clean for pictures, Mary came to set flowers about the house and decorate... and me? I'm just in my glory. I keep gazing at my breathtaking wedding gown. It hangs on my closet door just as my first prom gown did sixteen years ago. Mom and Dad look so incredibly happy. And I'm incredibly ecstatic. I've never been so excited in my whole life. I feel wonderful!

October 9, 1994

Couldn't sleep a wink last night. I just stirred, tossed, and turned. I swear someone slipped a pea underneath my mattress! I couldn't get comfortable. Now I can hardly write, my hands are shaking so. It's time to get ready for the ball!

Something borrowed, nothing blue. I feel like a real princess!

October 11, 1994

MRS. BARBARA DOOLING! BARBARA DOOLING! BARB DOOLING! DOOLING, DOOLING, DOOLING!!! A prince and princess were carried off in a Cinderella carriage! Mom and Dad rode with

Barbara Dooling

me in the carriage from their house to the church. Then Mr. and Mrs. Thomas Dooling sipped Champagne in the carriage and the horse trotted off as we waved to everyone. Yes, it truly was a "royal" wedding. We really were carried off by a white horse and a white carriage just as the story books foretold. Although the wedding was not elaborate and expensive, it was exceptional just because it was ours! I'm writing this on the plane while we're jetting off to paradise—Hawaii!

Back to the wedding…

I was radiant! I wore a lace ivory gown entirely beaded with sequins. It shimmered like sun on sand and glimmered like the moon on water. The train was cathedral length with scalloped edges. The bodice had tiny buttons down the back, and the front was covered by a sheer mesh neckline that was fitted with strands of pearls which dangled to my bosom. The wedding gown was stunning and I felt like a real princess. My veil met the length of the train. The crown was a simple Juliet cap with sequins and lace roses. My bouquet was small and delicate with white roses and three white orchids. I used the same thick ivory satin ribbon from Mom's bouquet—something old. The bride's maids wore burgundy velvet full, length gowns. Each had a long slit up the back of the skirt. The neckline was accented with ivory lace and sequins. They were elegant!

The nuptial mass was celestial. We were married in St. Mary's Church in Dedham where I had been baptized and had attended mass my whole life. It is a most beautiful old brick cathedral with an ornate white marble altar that resembles a fancy wedding cake. Dad walked me down the aisle slow and steady. I thought I might cry from so much happiness, but I beamed with the grandest smile and nodded gracefully to all our guests as I passed them in the

Impossible Choices

pews. Nearing the altar, my eyes met Tom's gaze. He looked dashing in his tuxedo. Tom never took his eyes off me until Dad extended my arm to him to give me away.

Our reception hall was adorned with lovely Victorian decor. We had the ceramic wedding boots filled with roses neatly centered on round mirrors with two white candles flickering soft light, and wavering a reflection into the glass. Our cake resembled a white gazebo, laced with burgundy ribbon and roses. And a Victorian boot stood on either side of it. I didn't have my Angel on top because Carolyn let us borrow the decoration that she had on her own wedding cake. It's a blown glass heart with two wedding bells dangling inside. The wedding party was introduced from a high staircase in the center of the hall. Then the prince and princess descended with guests cheering and smiling. I could see their eyes fixed on my shimmering gown as I took each step, guided by my new husband. I did feel like Cinderella at the ball as we stepped onto the parquet floor and glided to a waltz for our first dance as Mr. and Mrs. Thomas Dooling. At that moment, I was certain that I was the happiest woman in the whole world.

Dad even got to dance to Daddy's Little Girl with me! I had to finally break down then! I was slightly taller than Dad. As I wept, my tears rolled onto his black tux. I whispered, "I love you, Daddy" and the two of us were crying like babies. If that didn't make me cry enough, Tom and I each danced with our siblings to the song *Wind Beneath My Wings*. We started the song off dancing together. Then, since he has four sisters and I have four brothers, we had the DJ call each sibling up to the dance floor to cut in. I included Bruce in the dance as well. Now it seemed that everyone was crying. What a crew!

Tom and I had our going away dance together before I presented my bouquet to my matron of honor, Mary. We waltzed again, this time to what other than... *Beauty and The Beast*. He didn't step on my toes once, nor I his. We had taken dancing lessons before the wedding and practiced many evenings on the kitchen floor after working for hours painting those wedding boots. My going away outfit was an elegant ivory dress and jacket with Satin and sequins bordering the collar. After detaching the veil, I kept my Juliet cap on which became a lovely hat. Again, I felt beautiful.

October 21, 1994

Our honeymoon in romantic Hawaii has been filled with sensational sunny days and sensuous loving nights! The newlyweds shared love and made love for two weeks in dreamland Maui! Today is our last day here on this paradise island. I can only keep repeating to myself that I've never been happier in my life. Tom is the kindest, most sincere man I have ever known. This was a marvelous beginning to our wonderful life together. My head is still whirling with delight. I love him. I am sooooo in love with him. I have found my soul-mate!

In between site seeing, we relaxed on these glorious beaches. Luscious green mountains jut out of the ocean. We've sat from sunup to sundown with that sensational view... reading, snoozing, picnicking, playing and kissing. By now, we're both deep bronze. Today I sit on the open balcony at the condo we rented; we're both brooding because our vacation is over—but not the honeymoon! Anyway, it's been a grand time.

Reminiscent of these golden days, we took in a Luau where we saw Hawaiians dance with fire, while beautiful women swung their hips back and forth so fast you'd swear they popped their joints. Their grass skirts rustled to the beat of drums. For our dinner, a pig

Impossible Choices

was roasted in the ground beneath huge green leaves. I didn't think I could eat that hog because its head, snout and eyes kept popping into my mind. But that meat looked so juicy and tender I made myself try it. It was scrumptious.

Tom managed to talk me into a helicopter ride. I was reluctant because I've heard they sometimes crash into the high mountains. He said we'd make great headlines back home: newlywed couple perish in copter crash! Very funny, Tom. I did get on that chopper and I absolutely loved it! We flew above the ocean, close to the cliffs. Between the water and the rolling slopes I never saw so many shades of green. The elevation made my ears pop and we glided in and out of a volcano so quickly that my stomach did a flip-flop like the day Tom asked me to marry him. Suddenly, it began to rain. I was so bummed that the weather was uncooperative on our first helicopter ride. But the pilot told me not to fret because it was going to be a sensational ride now that it was pouring. All at once, the mountains were gushing with hundreds of waterfalls. Oh, how breathtaking it was! Just amazing! I was actually crying because I was so overwhelmed. If that wasn't wonderful enough, the rain stopped, the sun peeped through and out jumped a gorgeous double rainbow! Imagine a double! At that moment, I was screaming and crying. I think the pilot was concerned I might jump out and try to fly myself "somewhere over that rainbow." I kept yelling to Tom, "Look how beautiful. My God, Look at it, Tom. Oh, look, look, look!" He gripped my hand tightly and said, "I'm looking, I'm looking." And he kissed me quickly so we wouldn't lose a second of that site. I'll never forget that moment as long as I live!

Before the two weeks were over, we took a private sailing cruise out to a coral reef to go snorkeling, drove the winding road to Hana, and watched a brilliant sunrise on top of the volcano,

Barbara Dooling

Haleakala—elevation, 9,740 feet! There was dancing every night in the loveliest Hotel lounges, Black Sand Beaches, and shopping at downtown Lahaina. I don't think there was a thing we missed on this island. Tomorrow we fly out of here… no wonder we're moping!

December 25, 1994

We are still living at Big Tom and Al's. We woke today to an empty house. My dear sweet mother-in-law dragged poor Donna out of bed at the crack of dawn, and the three of them snuck down to Tricia's for breakfast. Tom and I had our first "married" Christmas in private thanks to Alice. We sat on the oriental living room rug beneath the "Dooling" tree that Al let ME decorate! I used many of my own ornaments, mixed with hers. It's a lovely tree. What a kind gesture since I found myself a newlywed in her home. It's been an adjustment for everyone, but Mom and Dad Dooling have made great efforts to make me feel comfortable. Today tops it off like the star on this tree.

February 11, 1995

Came up to Maine this weekend, an early celebration for Tom's birthday. Needed some time alone with my new husband. I surprised him with an exotic bouquet of tropical flowers like the ones we saw every day on our honeymoon. I ordered the spray from a florist in Boston and picked them up before the ride up. It's huge: Birds of Paradise, ginger, orchids, Anthurium, Heliconia, and Calla lily. It's a perfect arrangement for a guy because the flowers are so unusual. Tom is delighted. The bright orange and purple petals of the Birds of Paradise are very pointy like a bird's beak and head plumage. We hope to see several blooms come out over the next

Impossible Choices

few days. I remember Dad telling me that these plants can take up to five years to produce their first flowers. (I guess paradise is all about patience.)

The ginger root is a pink, sweet fragrant, and firm flower. Purple Dendrobium orchids cascade here and there with their delicate bells and sacs. While we were in Hawaii, Tom and I learned that these spectacular blossoms symbolize love, tenderness, friendship, and joy. That's every bit of our relationship all right! Anthurium which means tall flower in Greek, are shiny heart shaped petals of red, orange, pink, coral, and white. The Heliconia are just as tall and the florist said these are pollinated by hummingbirds! Their flowers are bright red with yellow tips. And the Calla lily are simple but lovely, the purest of white. Thank God I brought my own vase for these magnificent, bold, vibrant flowers because there is nothing at the cottage that would hold them! Wow… they are just gorgeous.

March 17, 1995

How good it was to get away last month! It's been five months since we moved in with Tom's parents. It's weird to be here. Tom is perfectly at home of course, since this was his home and these are his folks. But for me, let's not forget that I've been living on my own for fifteen years with one quick pit stop back to Mom and Dad's when I returned from California. Here I am, a newlywed living with Alice, big Tom, and Donna. I will say that Al and big Tom go to Maine frequently which gives us some privacy. Tom should feel fortunate though, I've adjusted to these living arrangements very well. And I'm very friendly with his family. I can't see him living at Mom and Dad's—no way.

So Tom is perfectly content because we are really able to save our pennies while searching for our own home. I am grateful for my in-laws' generosity. Believe me, they've gone overboard in making me feel welcome. I have no horror in-law stories. My mother-in-law couldn't be nicer. And I'm sure they've had to adjust to us being here, too. Okay, so the most difficult thing for me is making love to Tom with Tom's parents in one room and his sister in the other, and us in the middle! I'm just mortified! A brand new bride... and my groom gets aroused by the mere sight of me, he's always ready willing and able to fool around. I need only brush by him and he's stimulated, ready to hit the sack at eight o'clock. Hmmm, I wonder why Barb and Tom have gone up to bed so early? Oh God, I'm beside myself! To make matters worse, our bedroom door doesn't close properly. There is a small crack, which to me might as well be as big as the Grand Canyon. I hang my bathrobe and try to shove the material through the crack. I must be paranoid. As if someone is going to peek inside! But I just can't stand it. So, when Tom's parents head to Maine again, he promised me that he would take the door off the hinges and try to fix it.

I also feel funny cooking in Al's kitchen. Two women in the same kitchen is like two elephants in a galley. But Al and I do pretty well. Again, I'm easy going and so is she. Al basically does the cooking because I don't get home from work until six. Not a bad deal having dinner on the table when you get home from a hectic day at the office. But sometimes I'd like to cook for my husband. Although I will say that having dinner ready allows us to go out on appointments, looking for houses. I thank my lucky stars we are living here rent free so we can save more for a down payment. But after all these years of waiting—my mind and heart finally in sync— yet I still can't totally let go to enjoy my lover. I can't wait to make all the noise I want when I'm having sex with my husband! And I can parade around in a sexy nighty, or better yet, naked. Have a

Impossible Choices

quickie in the afternoon, and a longie at night. To linger in bed on Sunday mornings kissing, loving, and feeding each other with pleasure. I want to leave naughty notes on his pillow, but I dare not! Tom is so comfortable and nonchalant that he eases my anxiety. Still, I just can't wait to get our own place.

July 23, 1995

After eight months living with Tom's parents, we bought our modest three bedroom colonial in Melrose. Thank heavens for Tom's wonderful mom and dad! They've been more than generous! Our home is our castle. I had always wanted a Victorian house, but it's no matter. I'll make that dream come true by getting a Victorian dollhouse someday for the little girl or (girls) we'll have! Tee Hee.

After spending countless weekends looking at homes in various towns, we finally joined the homeowners' club. Tom and I have been working side-by-side evenings and weekends, renovating our new home. We do yard work, scraping, painting, and repairing—none of which have ever been any hobbies of ours. I didn't realize what a handyman I married, and I've surprised myself at what I can do. I've become quite the apprentice.

We've been content spending our summer putting our personal touches. There were many boxes to unpack… plenty of junk, stuff, things—his, mine, and ours. We tried to compromise on what stayed and what got thrown into the "yard sale pile." There was much negotiating since we both had had our own apartments before we got married. Our paraphernalia differed greatly in style and taste.

October 15, 1995

We celebrated our first anniversary at Disney World in Florida.

Barbara Dooling

As many times as I have been there, it never ceases to transform me into a child again. We returned to the comforts of our new home. Autumn has come with its pleasant aromas and splendid display of bright colors: scarlet red, lemon yellow, salmon, and bronze. We spend our free days apple picking, carving pumpkins, horseback riding, and wearing bulky wool sweaters to football games. The squirrels have been getting plump round bellies, bushy tails, and thick fur coats. They can be seen feverishly gathering nuts underneath our oak tree out back. I love to watch them chase each other around the wide trunk. I am content beyond words with this life of ours.

December 29, 1995

The Thanksgiving and Christmas holidays were bountiful—filled with joy and laughter of family and close friends. Cool breezes and crisp fall evenings have given way to frigid air and bare motionless trees. There is no stopping the seasons. Cozy and safe inside our lovely new home, we watched the beginning of winter display a blustery storm. It was a deep snow, concealing the very tips of our miniature evergreens in the front yard. The newly planted azalea bushes were completely hidden. Despite its heaviness, the snow was silent as it fell to the ground. It always amazes me how those delicate flakes can accumulate so. It is truly a winter wonderland.

April 1, 1996

I'm pregnant!

April 10, 1996

Though the weather has been changing and misleading these past few weeks, spring has finally arrived. We all like this season to

Impossible Choices

be punctual, but I do not think Mother Nature has a calendar. With warmer days comes the promise of blossoms, beginning with the brave crocuses forcing their way through the frozen ground. Next, tiny buds on the trees and bushes begin to sprout. Purple and pink rhododendron and sunshine yellow forsythia follow suit. We've had spring fever, Tom and I. We've been taking long walks together getting to know our neighborhood. On April Fools' Day I strung pastel pink and blue balloons to the front porch. I tied two dozen in all and placed a banner on the door announcing to Tom that I was pregnant. When he came home from work that day, he said the balloons were blowing the news down the street. As soon as he turned the corner, he knew. The small bulletin placed on the front door was written with a poem. It read: "It's no joke, I'm not fooling, there soon will be another Dooling!" Once inside, Tom jolted me off my feet and swung me around! More dreams are coming true! Can a person be this happy? I'm thirty-five and I'm going to have a baby!

On Easter Sunday, we made the rounds with our big announcement. I arrived with my usual white, wicker basket with colored eggs filled with goodies. Only this year, there was no candy inside! I sealed each one of those eggs with a special message. There the basket sat perched proudly on the table... center stage just waiting for someone to select an egg. I was so excited! Tom hurried his mom and dad along, offering them one of those treats. At my parent's house, mom and dad cried!

August 17, 1996

I have loved every moment of my plump belly; it is just like a basketball. Tom says I don't even look pregnant from behind. I feel tremendous and healthy. I've lots of energy and I still run up the stairs two at a time. Everyone, especially Mom, is telling me to slow

Barbara Dooling

down. I've had more advice than a psychiatrist can give from every woman whose ever had a baby. And the best advice has come from those women who've never had a baby...

Ha! I'm to keep my feet up (but I don't have swollen ankles), sleep on my left side (as if I could sleep on my stomach anyway), get plenty of sleep (as if anyone could sleep with a basketball... one that's constantly bouncing), and lord knows a million other tips. Those are the Do's. The Don'ts are: Don't stretch your arms over your head (but how do I hang clothes and wash my hair?), don't have sex (but... but... but...), and don't put anything in the house for the baby; it's bad luck. Now that one really got me mad. As if having a crib ready for the baby is going to give it a birth defect. The way I figure it, if our baby is born with Down's syndrome or has a birth defect, he or she is still going to need a crib. Heaven forbid the baby dies, our grief will be no more or less if there's a crib to put in storage. I won't say who, but I had someone act very concerned for the baby because I had put a few baby bottles in the cabinet. Everyone is entitled to their own opinion, but why would anyone want to upset a pregnant lady? I guess I wasn't all that upset since the bottles are still there. Oh yah, I'm going to have a boy because I'm carrying low. Or was that a girl because my birth date plus my due date are an even number.

September 8, 1996

The nursery is ready! It looks adorable. We've decorated it in classic Winnie The Pooh. Pooh and his friends—Tigger, Rabbit and Roo are everywhere! The dark cherry crib has a canopy with a matching dresser and changing table. What a sensational room! The baby will sleep in a cradle in our room for a few months, but his or her room is ready! I love standing in that room and staring at the

Impossible Choices

huge stuffed Pooh bear that Bruce gave us. We put Pooh in the crib! Tom catches me daydreaming and wraps his arms snugly around me and our baby. He nestles his face in the crook of my neck and gives me a sensuous kiss. We're paying no attention to those warnings about no sex!

September 21, 1996

Baby and I danced this day away at my niece Kim's wedding. My tummy is quite big and round, but I had no trouble kicking up my feet on the dance floor. What a splendid day Tom and I had! He told me I looked radiant! I felt pretty in the lovely green maternity dress with a lace collar. I bought it especially for the wedding. Of course the bride is always the star on the day she gets married, but Tom made me feel as stunning as Kim.

October 6, 1996

Mary and all my maids from the wedding gave me a baby shower today. Everything was decorated with Winnie including a Pooh bear sitting in an upside down umbrella on the cake. I laughed so hard when I saw the favors: bear shaped bottles of honey! How appropriate! Of course bears love honey, especially Pooh. What a delightful afternoon and we got lovely gifts! My basketball is really round and inflated. I never took off my shoes. Mom says a lady never takes off her shoes. I giggled and wiggled and this baby's still rumbling in my tummy. Now with all these generous toys, clothes, carseats, a high chair, and a stroller we're ready for Kyle Thomas or Kara Elizabeth.

November 18, 1996

Introducing... Kara Elizabeth Dooling!!!! She's here, she's here,

Barbara Dooling

she's here!! This is the most amazing day of my life!

November 21, 1996

EXTRA, EXTRA READ ALL ABOUT ME

STORK DELIVERS: Male Female ***
Calf Chick Cub Cherub Colt Child***

MY PARENTS ARE BARBARA AND TOM DOOLING:
Proud*** Ecstatic*** Boasting***
All Of The Above***

MY NAME IS LITTLE MISS KARA ELIZABETH DOOLING.
I ARRIVED TWO WEEKS EARLY BY SURPRISE:
Cesarean Section Parcel Post
Certified Mail Special Delivery***

NOVEMBER 18, 1996 AT 3:38am,
WEIGHT 5 lbs 11 oz, AT A SPAN OF 18 1/2
Yards Feet Inches*** Kilometers Meters

I AM JUST A BUNDLE OF:
Nerves Groceries Joy*** Wood

MY HAIR IS:
Black Brown*** Blonde Red No Hair

IT LOOKS LIKE:
Peach Fuzz*** Lion's Mane Curly Clown

Impossible Choices

MY EYES ARE: Blue   Green   Brown***

I HAVE VERY PETITE FEATURES
AND EVERYONE SAYS I LOOK LIKE:
My Mommy***   My Daddy   The Mailman

BUT MOMMY SAYS I HAVE DADDY'S EYEBROWS AND HIS:
Dimple***   Pimple   Beard

I AM JUST SO CUTE THAT MOMMY AND DADDY SAY
THEY ARE GOING TO:
Drop Me   Keep Me***   Trade Me

EVEN THE NURSES IN THE HOSPITAL THINK
I'M ADORABLE AND TINY.
I HAVE A ROOMMATE IN THE NURSERY WHO IS A HUGE 12lb:
Turkey   Baby Boy***   Roast

THE NURSES PLAY AND LAY US SIDE BY SIDE
TO COMPARE OUR:
Sizes***   Blankets   Parents

LABOR AND DELIVERY WENT EXTREMELY FAST.
AT 9:30 pm ON SUNDAY NIGHT MOMMY'S WATER BROKE.
THE DOCTOR SAYS THE MEMBRANES RUPTURED.

MOMMY HAD NO LABOR PAINS. DADDY WENT BACK TO:
Work   Bed***   Drawing Board

Barbara Dooling

HE KEPT HIS CLOTHES ON TO BE READY FOR THE GREAT:
Escape   Escort   Arrival   Departure***

BY 12:30 am, MOMMY SAID:
It's Time***   Good Grief   Good Night   Good Riddens

THEN AWAY WE: Flew   Drove***   Galloped

DADDY WENT STRAIGHT TO THE:
Mall   Airport   Hospital***

NO ONE WOULD BELIEVE I WAS MOMMY'S FIRST BABY
BECAUSE LABOR WAS STEADY AND CONTRACTIONS WERE
ALREADY FOUR MINUTES APART AT 1:30 IN THE MORNING.

LUCKILY THERE WAS A:
Chef   Teacher   Lawyer   Doctor***

HE WAS RIGHT THERE ON:
Board   Campus   Call***

THIS JUST HAPPENED TO BE MOMMY'S OWN PHYSICIAN.
UNFORTUNATELY, MOMMY HAD BEEN EATING SPICY FOOD
ALL WEEKEND WHICH GOT ME DOING:
Backflips***   Tummersaults***   Cartwheels***
All Of The Above***

I MUST HAVE TURNED AROUND IN HER BELLY AND
MY HEAD GOT STUCK UNDER HER RIB CAGE
SO THE DOCTOR HAD TO TAKE ME BY C-SECTION.

Impossible Choices

MOMMY WAS AWAKE THROUGH THE WHOLE OPERATION. DADDY GOT TO BE IN THE:
Classroom   Kitchen   Garage   Operating Room***

HE WATCHED THE GREAT:
Procedure***   Stunt   Battle   Performance

I CAME OUT: Screaming***   Sleeping   Laughing

BOTH MOMMY AND DADDY:
Cried***   Laughed***   Kissed***
All Of The Above***

DADDY HELD ME TIGHTLY. HE LOVED ME AND KISSED ME BEFORE HE HANDED ME OVER TO MOMMY.

WE ARE A REAL FAMILY NOW:
The Adams Family   The Von Trapp Family
The Dooling Family***

December 20, 1996

Kara is so small that we fit her into a Christmas stocking and placed her underneath the tree. Our first Christmas together as a little family was quite typical, I imagine. We adore our new daughter! We have been beaming with pride. The evenings have gotten much shorter since our newly imposed bedtime. Our little one is still not sleeping through the night—waking at least three times before dawn. It's early to bed, early to rise. Tom and I have a lot of pillow talk. It's our special time together. When I nurse Kara Elizabeth, Tom watches over my shoulder with such contentment. Our life is joyous. We are elated. We are living the fairy tale—happily ever after!

January 11, 1997

How delightful our Christmas was with this blessed addition to our family. I am the happiest I have ever been. Can life be any than this? Kara Elizabeth is a miracle. (I guess every birth is a miracle.) She sleeps soundly swaddled tightly in a Winnie the Pooh receiving blanket in a wooden cradle that Tom slept in. I pull that cradle closer to my bedside every night. I must put my pen down for a moment to gaze at her tiny body. A white stocking cap with a pink bow fits snugly on her head. All I can see is a tiny rounder-than-round face with a teensy button nose and the most perfectly shaped soft pink lips. I want to scoop her up, take off all the bundles, and munch on her flesh! My mouth waters for baby meat!!!

January 18, 1997

Kara is eight weeks old! Tom's Uncle Howard, who is a Deacon, Christened her today during a private ceremony. She wore the ivory lace gown that has been passed down since Russ wore it fifty years ago. The gown is outfitted with an ivory satin jacket that Mom Dooling ironed, and the material shines like new. Uncle Howard used a conk shell from the Caribbean beaches to anoint Kara's head with water from the font. During her baptism, she gazed up at the dim lights that twinkled above the marble altar. She was content and mesmerized. Our family and friends gathered to witness our precious baby being welcomed into the church. Tom and I stood proudly. I was crying soft, happy tears. The seashell made me think of the ocean where it came from—where we all came from. It is

Impossible Choices

water that sustains life; we come from water in our mother's womb. I shall save the white shell with its bright pink smooth middle coiled up inside. It will be a wonderful keepsake for Kara.

February 22, 1997

The three Dooling bears hibernate for a few days at Grammy and Grampy's cottage in Maine. This weekend is Tom's thirty-fourth birthday. He claims that he has everything he wants...a beautiful wife... a precious baby girl... and a wonderful life. Oh it is a wonderful life... it really is! My happiness is boundless. I could explode with joy. Tom gets a fire going in the wood stove and I settle Kara Elizabeth in my arms. I cannot seem to put her down. It is no great wonder how babies get spoiled. I love to hold her and watch her sleep. She and the flames in the stove warm me. Kara awakes with a hungry cry and turns her head toward me in search of my breast. I offer her my engorged bosom; she suckles with the strength of a lion cub. Ouch, what a barracuda. Tom is aroused by this Norman Rockwell scene. When she appears to have filled her small belly, the breast is dry, and she drifts back to sleep. Tom steals the babe from my clutch and returns her to the porta-crib. He promises to be more gentle on my breasts than our daughter, and we lay right there in front of the warm blaze and turn Rockwell into Harlequin. Happy Birthday, Daddy, Tom.

April 26, 1997

For my own birthday celebration, we take Kara to Maine, but this time we splurge and spend one night at the Anchorage Inn in Ogunquit. The evening is spent splashing in an outdoor Jacuzzi while Kara sleeps alongside in her car seat. She is bundled up warm and we throw a blanket over her to protect her from the night air.

Barbara Dooling

Our days and nights together as a new family are filled with much love. These small getaways are such a treat. We just finished taking a nice hot shower (together) since we nearly froze our fannies off during the mad dash to get back to the hotel room. Again, we brought Kara with us! She remained sleeping in her seat on the bathroom floor while we lathered each other up... and more. I kept peeking out of the shower curtain to make sure she was still breathing. What can I say, except I'm a paranoid new mother. Tom surprised me with a pear shaped diamond necklace! It is lovely and matches my engagement ring. We cannot afford such luxuries, but I will not ruin his splendid gift with such talk. Tomorrow we head up a few exits to Old Orchard. The remainder of the weekend will be spent at the cottage. As for tonight, it isn't over yet! The fun has just begun! Happy 36th Birthday to me!

May 7, 1997

What a fairy tale I am living. I'm in total awe! I am so in love with Tom and so completely elated with our baby girl Kara. Tom and I cuddle her up between us and talk softly into the night until we doze ourselves. I know, I know, it is the absolute worst habit... everyone warns not to do it, but we love to nestle Kara Cub between us in the big bed. Before I had her, I swore I'd never let my children sleep with us! For one thing, if Kara is having a tough night with gas or colic at two o'clock in the morning, all rules go out the window! Whatever quiets her down is what we do! Second, there is nothing so precious as laying peacefully with a sleeping baby snuggled to your chest. How do I explain the joy it gives to me watching our baby sleep. She is truly a precious jewel. Her sweet smell comforts me. Those teeny tiny little fingers that stretch into the air amaze me, and the cooing and murmur sounds she makes

Impossible Choices

stirs something inside of me that is indescribable. Tom gazes at his two "girls" with such pride it always makes me misty eyed.

She is six months old and sitting up and crawling—crawling backward no less! It is amusing to watch her get stuck against the couch because she can't see where she's going. Do babies actually crawl backward? I keep putting toys in front of her to encourage forward motion. She is not at all interested in going after that rattle. Instead she puts her small self in reverse and creeps until she bangs into furniture. That must come from Tom's side.

May 11, 1997

A toothy! Bear Cub has a toothy! I see a tiny bud poking through her pink gums! Tee hee hee hee! A tooth! And on my first Mother's Day no less!

June 14, 1997

Her nickname suits her! She growls like a bear, too. She has found her voice. Kara Cub growls when she eats, plays, and even in her sleep. It's hysterical. Grrrrrr, Grrrrrr, Grrrrrr!

July 10, 1997

I don't think that this is actually my hand writing these words tonight... surely it must be someone else's... for it seems like it would be impossible for it to be my own hand. Surely the phone didn't really ring, and those weren't my ears hearing Dr. Jeff say, BREAST CANCER... surely he didn't tell ME that I was the one with cancer. Cancer? See, that's not my hand writing that dark demon word on the beautiful white clean hopeful pages of my journal. It couldn't be me he wanted to see in his office right away—TODAY if I could manage it. Were those really my legs that walked out of that doctor's office a few hours later, and climbed into the car and drove all the way home without getting into a wreck?

This is all a terrible mistake… a bad dream… and I will wake in a few hours, and everything will be sunny again. My hands are shaking—look at my penmanship—these words are jagged and spilling over the lines on the page. I'm in a panic here because I know in my heart that this is NOT a dream. That's right; I can actually feel my heart pounding right through my chest. This is real and I can't escape it… I can't breath… My life has changed forever. Oh, please don't let it be true… please oh please, oh please. My fairy tale is over and the nightmare has just begun… Cancer… Breast Cancer, there must be a mistake. How? Why? What caused it?

My precious Kara, only eight months old, sat on the living room floor while the doctor spoke. Kara's sweet yet strong voice bellowing her happy talk, "daaaah daaaah daaaah, mum mum mum, eeeeh eeeeh, baaaah baaaah." I hung up the phone and scooped her into my arms and held her close to my heart for comfort. She was the only one at home. As I cradled her, I just sobbed and kissed her soft, tender, tiny cheek. She began to struggle and pull away because I was squeezing her so tightly and covering her with kisses. We circled the downstairs rooms pacing the floor over and over again. I couldn't sit still; I couldn't concentrate. I couldn't do much of anything. Finally, I returned Sweetie Girl to her activities while I sat in my own silence.

I haven't finished her baby book!! I should have put those millions of pictures into her album. My whole day is a blur now. My mind took off full-speed, faster than I could keep up, hurdling from one thought to the next. What special woman… just who would be a mother to this beautiful child of mine if something should happen

Impossible Choices

to me? What fine woman will love her as I do? Will she tell Kara everyday that she loves her? Will she show as much enthusiasm when Kara staggers with her first steps? Will she rock my baby girl in her arms and twirl her hair as my own mother did to me? Who will plan her birthday parties? Will she save every piece of my darling's art work? Will she teach my daughter to love animals like her mommy does? Who will guide her through those difficult adolescent years? Will this caring woman share secrets when Kara turns sixteen and when she is first kissed? What special lady will teach her about being a woman? Will she ensure that Kara learns to love and respect herself so that men and others will do the same? All of these questions and more ravished my brain.

After this moment of processing, I jumped up and grabbed the phone to call Tom. I was fairly calm as I broke the news to him—I only cried a little bit. He was stunned. There was this long pause of sucked in air. I wasn't even sure if he was still there on the other end of the receiver. Silence—pure silence. Poor Tom. He fled home from work right away. The minute he walked through the door, I melted in his arms. I was like a broken doll—could hardly stand up. As I sobbed on his shoulder, he said nothing. I know he was as scared as I was. We held each other all night long.

Mom and Dad were the next victims. Oh boy, they were weak with sorrow. Dad told me to have courage; Mom told me to have faith. They both told me they'd pray. Mary, Russ, Kenny, Paul, Geno... right on down the line. I called everyone. They all promised to help any way they could. Then Tom called his side: Mom and Dad, Margaret, Tricia, Carolyn, and Donna. No one can believe it! They all said I'm so young, no family history of breast cancer, it just can't be true—but it is true. It is indeed true! It's all too real. My God, it's all real. How am I going to hold back the ocean waves of cancer against my small self? Will I be a strong enough break wall?

When I finished calling the family, there was Sheila, Julie, and Bruce... Kim and Denise, my boss and everyone at work. Sheila and Julie cried so hard that they started me crying again. Bruce was despondent and quiet as usual. Kim, being a nurse, was full of information—important things. Denise lost an aunt whom she was very close with to breast cancer, so she was all tears too.

July 10, 1997

The phone hasn't stopped ringing. Neighbors, friends, and relatives are coming out of the woodwork with comforting words and offers for help. We are blessed, truly blessed with so many people who love us.

July 14, 1997

Today I went into work to tell my boss Andy—his eyes were filled with tears. I was touched by his genuine and heartfelt response. He even told me that he loves me. We've grown to be genuine friends these past three years. We're like partners in a business. I think this news has totally blown him away. And the girls! My secretary and Alison, our technician, have been truly moved by this news. Poor Alison, we call her The Kid, she is a kid. I'm like a big sister to her. She tells me that all the time! She's never had a sister. This is her first job since college and I've taught her the ropes. She's crushed—just overwhelmed. Alison is usually talkative and full of questions about Kara and our weekend. Monday mornings always begin with the lowdown about Alison and her roommates, some party they went to, or some new guy she's got a crush on. Then she settles up with me to hear all about my mommy-daddy-Kara happenings. Even amidst our morning routines of opening the

Impossible Choices

examining rooms, turning on the computers, copy machine, and retrieving the messages off the answering service, the rush of patients waiting to be checked in, and the telephone lines buzzing nonstop starting at 9:01, we manage to have a cup of Java and share grapevine talk. But sweet Alison could say nothing all day after I told her about the cancer. She is a very genuine and empathetic woman, and makes it seem that she feels as deeply about the news as I do.

July 15, 1997

Here I sit, still stunned. I'm only thirty-six—that's too young to die. Will I really have to come out of my fragile glass bubble? My dear sweet Tom, my love, my hero, and my very best friend... is he ready for what lies ahead? I know we're both thinking the worst and hoping for the best. We have to survive this, we just have to. I just have to! Who the heck will clean the darn toilet? Who will feed poor kitty? Who's going to keep the Tupperware cabinet arranged by shapes? What about that kitchen junk drawer? My mind is helter-skelter! How will my parents handle this? Will their own health be at risk from worrying about me? My dear, loving mother, does she deserve to bear these pains a mother feels for her child? After all, I am her baby; I feel so sorry for her. Does she deserve this heavy burden? Then there are the medical questions: How did I develop this disease? Where did it come from? What did I eat that could have contributed to it? Was it the environment? Was it hormones; what? Not even the best physicians in Boston have given me definite answers.

I'm dumbfounded at how little is known about breast cancer. Surely with modern science and state-of-the-art medical equipment improving over the years, we would know more. So why can't my questions be answered? I simply don't believe this and I work in the

Barbara Dooling

medical field. More and more people are being diagnosed with cancer every year and no one really knows why. It has only been speculated. How could it be that science has put a high tech computerized craft on Mars? This land rover—a toy truck as it appears to me—roams another planet by being controlled from earth. Why can't anyone tell me how I got this cancer so I can stop whatever has caused it?

July 16, 1997

Six days have passed. I can't stop crying. One moment I am in control, the next I am sobbing. Fear of our uncertain future pierces my brain at the oddest moments. These are nothing short of spontaneous panic attacks. The chemotherapy that might actually save my life could change things forever. It could bring on early menopause by destroying ovarian function. We so wanted to have another child. In fact, shortly before the cancer was found, we were planning to get pregnant again. Will I even need chemotherapy? I won't know until after the surgeon takes the tumor out in two more weeks.

I adore my little girl. I am thankful for our sweet daughter—grateful to have had her. I don't want her to be an only child. I pray to God to let her have a brother or sister to share her life with. I pray that I will not need chemotherapy. I know, I know, first things first. I must save my life! But I will be crushed if we are not able to have another child. How selfish of me, when there are so many infertile couples who would love to be given the chance to have just one baby!

July 28, 1997

The lumpectomy with axillary node sampling is scheduled on

Impossible Choices

August fourth. They will remove the malignant tumor along with some surrounding tissue to make sure they get all the cancer. Obtaining clean margins is crucial. Node sampling is to determine if the cancer has spread to the adjacent lymph nodes underneath the armpit. This additional procedure is done to help stage the cancer, which will aid a treatment plan. Originally, Tom and I both wanted the surgeon to perform a mastectomy. We thought it best to take the whole breast—even take both breasts—if that meant getting rid of the cancer.

How very cavalier we were about losing the breast providing I could have my life in return. Because the size of my tumor appears to be fairly small, the surgeon assured us that a mastectomy was not necessary. In my case, it was explained that a lumpectomy, followed by six weeks of daily radiation, would be just as effective. Putting our trust in the doctor, we'll proceed with the lumpectomy.

August 7, 1997

Well, the tumor is out! The evening before my surgery, I pulled out my old china angel from the dining room hutch. My dear April Angel! I carefully wrapped her in bubble paper and packed her for the hospital. I cannot have this surgery without her watching over me. When I showed her to my neighbor Mary, I pointed out the broken wing, laughing and saying it symbolized me with my damaged bosom. With comforting words, my good friend Mary replied, "It's okay, Barbara. We are all angels with only one wing and we cannot fly unless we embrace each other." I thought about this all day. I have many people to thank for helping me to fly. I have all my friends, my family, my husband, and my precious Kara… and I shall soar with only one wing just like I have in the past!

Barbara Dooling

August 11, 1997
The doctor found more cancer during the surgery. And the procedure of removing twenty-five lymph nodes under my arm revealed that the cancer had spread to the lymphatic system. The final diagnosis is high grade multi-focal poorly differentiated infiltrating ductal carcinoma. In layman's terms, the tumor is aggressive. It was only 1.1 centimeters, which I am told, is relatively small, but it was invasive and not contained. Had the tumor not spread, known as "in situ," it would have been much better. The good news is that only one of those twenty-five nodes was positive for spread of cancer. However, this compiled with the finding of abnormal smaller tumors surrounding the main tumor means I will need chemotherapy as well as the radiation. A common hormone receptor test determined that the tumor was not estrogen fed; therefore I will not be a candidate for the wonder drug, Tamoxifen.

August 12, 1997
Since the surgery, fear has taken hold of me again paralyzing my thoughts and every inch of my body. I keep thinking of how I have heard people get sick from toxic side effects of the chemotherapy. I fear I will not be able to care for my baby. I don't want anyone else to take my place. I dread getting sick. Is this chemotherapy poison, or medicine? I hardly ever gave much thought to capital punishment by lethal injection, but I've been thinking about it lately. I have made myself sick to my stomach wondering about the toxicity of the chemotherapy. How truly amazing and powerful the mind is. I've decided that I will use this energy to help me fight this cancer—turning fear into hope.

Knowing that I do need chemotherapy has brought more unanswered questions and additional consultations with specialists. Not

Impossible Choices

only am I facing the disease, treatment, and recovering from surgery, but I am also dealing with preserving my fertility. This is a complication that post menopausal women with breast cancer are not faced with. In any event, pregnancy after breast cancer remains a controversial issue. Doctors have explained this is an area not well studied yet. The risks are considered theories.

If in fact we want to even consider the possibility of a future pregnancy, we have to remember that chemotherapy could impact my fertility. One recommendation is egg retrieval before starting on the chemotherapy. Hormones would be given by injection to stimulate more follicles which grow into eggs. Once the eggs are mature, they would be retrieved from the ovary and mixed with Tom's sperm to form embryos. The embryos would be frozen until we decided to become pregnant. But several doctors we've consulted feared that the hormones used to stimulate the ovaries to produce more eggs could trigger "some cancers." There seems to be no hard evidence and we found quite a discrepancy between opinions. Furthermore, since the procedure is done in conjunction with a menstrual cycle, this would also delay cancer treatment for at least one month. The ball is in my court and I'm not that great at tennis! We have little time to make our difficult decision.

August 15, 1997

Today I saw yet a different specialist who offered another option. This included an injection of Lupron, a drug often used to treat men with prostate cancer. In my particular case, Lupron works by suppressing the pituitary gland from releasing the female hormones which bring on menstruation. The use of Lupron for this purpose is somewhat new. It would basically shut the ovaries down, putting them to sleep. Therefore, if the ovaries are not trying to function they remain dormant during chemotherapy. They'll hopefully resume function with normal ovulation once treatment is completed. There's no real assurance that my periods would return, and it, too comes with its side effects. But since this course seems far less risky in relation to the cancer, this is the option we will pursue.

August 17, 1997

My niece Kim sent me a huge homemade card filled with messages using different pieces of candy. How clever. What a doll. And my boss Andy sent a huge flowering plant! Greeting and prayer cards from relatives and friends have been filling our mailbox daily. Tom has kept fresh cut roses of every color on the kitchen table. When they get the least bit wilted, he replaces them. I've received so many angel trinkets and statues that we had to buy a shelf because I now have a collection. The food and precooked dishes overflow from the frig and freezer. We have enough to start a restaurant. People have been so good to us. Tom's mom and dad have baby-sat for Kara countless times during my doctor's appointments and the hospital stay. I'm glad Kara isn't getting passed around from one house to another. Mary and Mom have set up a schedule, and each will stay with us for a few days to help with laundry and whatever else they see fit. I'm sure mom will be dusting all my furniture and keeping my plants watered. How lucky can one person be to have so much help pouring in?

August 18, 1997

Back to work today after two weeks recovering from the lumpectomy. I feel great, and I'm glad to be back in the swing of things. I could have taken more time off, but as long as I don't get

Impossible Choices

sick on the chemotherapy, there's no reason to. I hope and pray I don't.

September 25, 1997

Began chemotherapy. Cytoxan and Adriamycin at the end of August, just three weeks after the breast surgery. I really did much better than I ever imagined. With all the anxiety I had, I don't know how I ever showed up for the grand affair, but I did. To my surprise, I tolerated the chemotherapy quite well. Tom and I were prepared for the worst, placing basins in just about every room in the house. I never did get sick. Bravo, yippee! Hooray! But my periods ceased immediately between the Lupron drug and the chemotherapy. And I have had terrific hot flashes day and night. I began to keep track of these steamy surges and realized they were coming persistently every hour, twenty-four hours a day. They're so severe that I become weak with each one. I get quite uncomfortable and my clothing becomes soaked with sweat. During the night, I lose much sleep. The spells have me whipping the blankets off then an hour later I wake with the chills. It's been cold this fall and I have already lost all my hair. During a hot flash, not only do I shed the bedding, but I pull off my night gown and head turban. Next thing, I'm searching the bed for them in the darkness. This game of strip and cover up goes on all night long. What a side show!

I had hoped to have the same luck about losing my hair as I did with not getting sick on the chemotherapy. Maybe, just maybe, I wouldn't lose it. Silly ol' me. This is just one of the sacrifices to cancer, but I was well prepared. I had purchased a prosthetic hair piece while I still had my own hair. I prepared mentally by telling myself it was better than losing an arm or leg. No big deal, the hair will grow back. However, the minute the stylist put a nylon sock

Barbara Dooling

over my head to cover and catch my hair for trying on wigs, my eyes filled with tears. But I did not allow them to spill onto my face. I tried to hold my breath and not speak, fearing I would lose control.

The wig I picked out is almost a perfect match to my own hair and looks quite natural. I was beginning to feel better already. Well, that is until my hair actually fell out. Right on target, about two weeks after my first dose of chemotherapy, my hair began to shed. I found strands on my desk at work. At home, when I showered, the hair fell out in clumps. Within two days, my hair was more than molting like a duck's feathers. Scattered bald patches now replaced my beautiful, thick, wavy locks. I really did look like a cancer patient.

How truly vain I was. How was it I was so ready to lose my breast, but I was having such a difficult time over my hair? Who am I kidding? Losing the breast would have been devastating. My good friend Annie, a hair stylist, completed the balding process by shaving off what patches of hair that remained. She was quite moved by the job she had to do. I felt the coolness of the room on my scalp. On the floor, my soft locks were scattered about. I shall never complain about a bad hair day again. Though my scalp took some getting used to, I sort of like my head. Tom says it's a pretty head quite round and without a scar or blemish. He rubs it often and makes wishes as though it were a crystal ball. Sometimes he holds me in a headlock and gives me knuckle noogies until I cry uncle. He never wants me to wear the wig at home. He continues to tell me how beautiful I am. His support and good humor gives me light, and leads me through this dark jungle.

Impossible Choices

October 6, 1997

Between the chemotherapy and the Lupron injection, I am not sure whether I'm actually in menopause. All I know is that I continue experiencing those heat strokes. Some woman call them power surges. They're just plain awful. They come without warning and far too often for my patience. I was told the hot flashes were more frequent and intense than a natural menopause because they were chemically induced. I can't be given hormone replacement therapy because women with breast cancer or even a history of it can't take estrogen. One minute I'm freezing because I have no hair and the next I'm ready to tear my clothes off. Well, thank heaven Tom takes full advantage of the latter.

November 12, 1997

It's the second week of November and I've finally completed the regimen of chemotherapy! I was given the rest of the month off before starting the radiation treatment. My body needs time to bring the blood levels back to normal before radiation. How happy I am to have this break. Kara will be turning one on November eighteenth and I want to have the energy to give her a dazzling party. I remember praying to God last July to just let me live long enough to hear my baby call out, "Mamma!" And here I am, planning her first birthday. Kara will have a Winnie The Pooh bear cake and matching decorations. We will have that party!

November 16, 1997

Today we had a grand celebration for the birthday girl. Our little house was packed with Kara's cousins and friends. Andrew and Kenny Jr. came all the way from Rhode Island; and of course there were Mary's two kiddo's—Christopher and Alicia. Geno and

Barbara Dooling

Karen's clan: Nick, Matt, Mikie, and Tyla. Can't forget Daddy's side—Brittany, Kevin, and Calle, Ryan, Devan, and Brendan. Whew! And last but not least, Kara's second cousins Arliya and Stephanie and all the mommies and daddies. With my eyes full of tears and everyone singing the birthday song, Kara and I blew out her birthday candle. After smushing cake all over her face and in her hair, we tore pretty wrapping paper off lots of presents! That was great fun! When the destruction of packages and bows was finished, we lined up outside to have a ride on a real pony. Yes, adding to the festivities was Gigi girl, a delightful auburn and chestnut bay. Kara and Mamma trotted together for her first pony. I cried happy tears as I held Kara tightly against me. The rest of the children squealed with laughter as they mounted that pony. What a happy, happy day!

My baby girl, Kara, cannot only say "Mamma," but she has already taken her first steps. I'm still here to witness that new toddler waddle! How I laugh when she picks up speed only to go crashing to the floor. Sometimes she manages to stay standing, but she ends up colliding with the furniture. Little Kara is amazed where her feet can take her. And I am equally amazed at her development.

December 2, 1997

December has crept up on us as it tends to do. But today my thoughts aren't focused on the happy holidays. Tomorrow I begin my radiation, and I'm just as anxious about this as I was about the chemo. The doctor told me fatigue was a major side effect. I've kept myself busy by decorating the house and putting up the Christmas tree early. I won't have fatigue ruin our joyful holiday. Now that everything is done and in place, I'm ready to begin radiation—not really.

Impossible Choices

Radiation? Don't we get covered up by a large heavy vest at the dentist so we don't get radiated during x-rays? Tom has tried to joke with me by saying he will use me as a night-light if I begin to glow. Am I really going to go through with this? I've had several sleepless nights like the one I had before starting chemo.

Lately, I've been reading about alternative medicine: herbs, vitamins, and all that jazz. Maybe I should try something else? Radiation. The word alone frightens me. I had to sign a form acknowledging that radiation can cause other cancers or damage the heart or lungs. Of course this is rare, but then so is breast cancer at my age. Are doctors curing people with this standard western medicine? I'm at one of the finest hospitals in the country, aren't I? Enough nonsense. I must follow through with what I've started.

December 3, 1997

More litter for my beautiful journal... yep, that's right, more garbage! Today was the day. Day one of radiation. The waiting area was packed with people of all ages. It appeared that three men had brain tumors: their heads had been shaven and they had Frankenstein like scars from some awful surgery. Other women wore turbans. I was adorned with my trusty wig. I was holding together quite well, despite the appearances of these fellow cancer patients. Yes, I was doing fine until I saw a young boy, about seven years old. He too was bald. But he was wearing a big smile as if he had just visited the North Pole. I knew that Santa was not behind the door he came out of. I broke down at the next sight of a little three year old girl who had a brain tumor. I thanked God then and there for my having breast cancer instead of my Kara having a brain tumor. What were these children doing there anyway? Shouldn't they be at a children's hospital? Why did I have to endure this? Hmmm... If these wee babes could do it, I most certainly should stop feeling sorry for myself.

December 17, 1997

It's that time of year—the merry holidays! I never knew a person could have more than one guardian angel. Truly God has sent many angels to me throughout my illness: Tom and Kara, dear relatives and friends—old and new. Tom and I have been blessed. We are forever grateful.

Precious Kara has been our greatest inspiration. The joy she gives us each day takes our thoughts off the heavy burdens of my health. We have tried to focus on her and the wonderful miracles of her development. I just love how she toddles. Yes, she resembles a wind-up toy which rocks side-to-side until it topples over. It is difficult not to laugh at these crash landings. We clap for her and shout, "Hooray for Kara!" Then Kara picks herself up and claps too.

I was so filled with emotion the day of her first birthday party—it was such a delightful day. Daddy took lots of pictures and video so Kara will have this memory of her special day. That pony was a big hit!

Kara's vocabulary is limited, but increasing. She still babbles on in her own language as if we understand what she is saying. Daddy has taught her to say hello to Santa. He deepens his voice and bellows; "Ho, ho, ho!" And Kara repeats, "Ho, ho!" Daddy tries to get her to say all three ho's. Maybe next year, Daddy. Tee hee, hee!

Our tree has thus far survived Kara! This year it is tied to the wall so it will not fall over if she tugs on a branch. At first she was so mesmerized by the glittering lights and shiny ornaments that she did not touch it. However, curiosity took hand and she pulled on

Impossible Choices

the lower branches, the garland and pretty toy-like items. Mommy does want her to enjoy the tree, but she can't seem to do that without touching. Poor little Kara.

The spirit of Christmas fills our home and our hearts despite the goings on with my treatment of breast cancer. Tom and I have given each other love and mutual support. We cling to what we have instead of wishing for what we don't have. And we've learned an awful lot this year. During this holy season we especially thank God for those who have been so good to us. I pray for renewed health and safety for my family and friends always!

January 6, 1998

It's already January 1998; the days seem to pass so quickly. Do I dare say Happy New Year? Of course I dare to, after all I'm still here! Lately, I seem to read everything I can find about breast cancer. I wonder when my time will be my own again. Indeed my newly imposed education is beginning to consume me. I really must put it all away for a while. I've learned quite enough for the time being and I need to get back to reading baby books. I must be there for my precious family. Yes, that's a much better way to spend my time.

I am a common person. I have done nothing spectacular with my life, but I am so happy with my life. My life is simple but truly bountiful. This small, modest home is indeed my castle. I adore my little Kara. She is petite and a great wonder. I cherish my family and friends who perhaps are without fame on a world scale, but they are certainly notable to me. And I love dear, sweet Tom. He may not be a bloodline prince, but he is sincerely the most royal man on the earth.

I have always been grateful for my good health. When I see a person or child with a handicap, I thank God for being me. I like to

Barbara Dooling

recite a little prayer for the afflicted. Sometimes I call that person to mind days later and genuinely feel empathy and admiration for him or her. I can honestly say that I always take time to stop and smell the roses. I behold the beauty around me. I dance in awe at the grand views of nature: the turquoise ocean, the emerald mountains, the yellow moon, and the silver stars... indigo skies and golden meadows, too. And I cherish the simple sight of an elderly couple holding hands, still in love. I smile watching a child clench a melting ice cream—such a treat. I cry at weddings, like a lot of people do. But do they cry when they see a child sitting on Santa's lap, grinning and hoping? Maybe... I sure do. And I cry when I see children at Disney World fearlessly running to their favorite character for a hug, a handshake, or an autograph! I feel so touched by these simple events that I fill up with happy tears. I did all this before I got cancer.

Remember my honeymoon in Hawaii? Tom and I saw rainbows nearly every day. Yes, I cried looking at every one of them. They were never routine, not for me. What a feeling I had; it was wonderful. Each rainbow was more delightful and exciting than the one before. I have been told by people that I live in a fantasy world, but these special things are in the real world. They are not make believe! I am so glad I see them even if others do not. And I will continue to see them, despite cancer. I shall teach Kara to see them. I must have faith and forget my negative thoughts. I wish I had unshakable faith like Mom has. All I need is courage. Suppose I could journey to Oz so the wizard can get me some courage? Yes, that's what I'll do. I shall leave this instant!

Oh how I've rambled on in these pages of my precious journal. Lest we remember though, it is adventurous and fun to do that sometimes, although the cancer is one adventure I'd not dare to

Impossible Choices

embark on. Albeit, I see clearly how fortunate I am to have so many people who love me. I am tired since I've started this mixed up entry composite of a sprinkle of this and some spicing of that. I must lay my pen down and rest a while.

January 13, 1998

Wow, we're so fortunate for the many people who continue to send their love. Pretty greeting cards wishing us more cheerful days fill our mailbox. My letter carrier must think I'm someone special. That's how folks have made me feel. Each day I open the mail, I can't help but cry. It's Water Works with plenty of tissues as I read all the lovely words. I can't even fit anymore cards on the buffet and I've resorted to the dining room table. What a collection... what support! The love and prayers have touched me so deeply; I am quite overwhelmed. Indeed, all the warmth and compassion has eased my anxiety through this most difficult time. Since my initial diagnosis of breast cancer in mid-July, we have received tender, comforting words and countless offers for help. How grateful we are to everyone for their assistance through this frightening ordeal.

Mom and Dad have always taught me to have faith and courage; courage, courage, and more courage. I hope that God hears my prayers, and my family and I can put all this behind us. God, if I do have a guardian angel, can you please send her to me... quickly?! Please have my angel to watch over Tom and I, and our little Kara, too! I'm even calling on my fairy godmother. Make me well again!

January 15, 1998

Mary calls me every day—sometimes twice in one day. She sends me the prettiest sister cards. She writes poems inside that always cheer me up. She's not bad at poetry! Even little Alicia sent

Barbara Dooling

a get-well card today. She included a class assignment for Martin Luther King Day. It's entitled: I Have a Dream, Too

Alicia writes:

I dream that there will be a cure for cancer because then my aunt will not be sick. If she dies, I will be really sad. She has a little girl. She will be really, really sad too. That is what my dream is. I can make my dream come true by becomig (spelled incorrectly) a docter and try to figure out a cure.

January 16, 1998

Last treatment of radiation! Yahoo! Yippee! Tom presented yellow and red roses with a card that read: *To Our Bright Future!* Oh, I hope so, Tom… I really and truly hope so. Dinner, champagne, and gold angel earrings followed those roses. That was celebration enough, but he had more up his sleeve with a single red rose left on my pillow. I must put my pen down for the best is yet to come. Our evening is just beginning.

January 20, 1998

I am forever told that I come from "good stalk" and a long line of hard working people with fine moral values. Boy, I sure could use some of that longevity and backbone to help me get through this! Mom was one of twelve children born in 1923 to a middle class Italian family. She always told me that her family was fortunate because during the depression they had good food to eat and warm clothes on their backs. Her father built a large home that housed her big family. Mom looks back on her childhood as "wonderful."

Dad was probably a little less lucky, but he still had parents who loved him. For some reason that I don't think I'll ever know, Dad lived with his maternal grandparents for most of his younger child-

Impossible Choices

hood. He was the eldest of four children, and when it came time for him to go back and live with his family again, he felt like an outcast. Dad says that his siblings thought he was trying to boss them around—he probably was. I can speculate that there was some jealousy because they had less attention, food, and toys, to go around than he did. He may have had a lot extra material things living at his grandparent's house, but he did not have his mother and father or his siblings! So he struggled to fit in, and did manage to have some kind of a family life.

I remember when Nana died at the age of ninety-seven, Dad told me he never knew why his mother "gave him up" as a baby. For him to mention this on the day his mother died, it must have been a deep-seeded issue. I suspect that dad carried that hurt with him all his life. Lord only knows if this was part of his drinking problem. That, and the fact that he was laid-off numerous times. It must have been a struggle raising the six of us children while being out of a job.

Mom and Dad were married in the fall of 1944. To this day, every time I look at their wedding picture, I wish I knew them when they were young. Without a doubt, they were the most beautiful couple. Dad was amazingly handsome and Mom was strikingly pretty. From the time I was a little girl, I always looked at that wedding picture and dreamed that I would someday be a beautiful bride like Mom, and marry a handsome man like Dad. Yep, I love their wedding pictures. Mom's gown was simple, but elegant. And dad wore his military uniform. They were a dream couple right out of the fairy tales.

After their military ceremony, Mom and Dad had one evening together before he was shipped over seas during World War II. Not much of a honeymoon, but they remained faithful to each other,

Barbara Dooling

and fortunately Dad returned from the war unharmed. I love snooping through the countless love letters from Dad that are inside Mom's hope chest. Years of memories are stored in that mahogany chest. There are flowers and ribbons, negligees, and greeting cards. Tiny baby clothes and a beautiful lace christening gown… yellowed envelopes labeled "Russell's and Kenny's first haircut." And wrapped inside the envelopes are soft locks of curly golden hair. More keepsakes are report cards and hand made cards; medals and honor ribbons. Yes, Mom's hope chest is filled with things that are worthless yet priceless. There are no gemstones, but there are many treasures. Now I have a hope chest and I've started filling it with dreams come true! But it's only half full! Pray for me, Mom… pray that I get to finish filling mine!

Even some of Dad's trophies are packed away in that cedar chest. During the late 1940's and 1950's, dad competed in the New England nationals for weightlifters. He weighed one hundred twenty-three pounds of solid muscle. In the light weight competition, dad placed second in 1947, third in 1949, and second in 1954. At the 1954 seniors, he cleaned and jerked a national record of two hundred fifty-six and a half pounds. It was double his body weight. He held this New England record in his lightweight division from the late forties into the fifties.

Dad was indeed a champion weightlifter. But, after he and Mom married, we came along and Dad had family obligations. His weight lifting career turned into lifting toddlers and scooters. (In 1993, he was inducted into the New England weightlifters' hall of fame at the age of seventy-five.) What an accomplishment! Hmm, I need some of that great strength. I really need that drive—that power! I had it back in high school on the track team. Got to get back into shape to fight this blasted cancer!

Impossible Choices

If there's anything I've learned over the years it's that all families have troubles, even some of those friends and relatives I went running to when I was young. I thought their lives were like the Brady Bunch, and that all their problems got solved in a half hour. Hah! Well, I know better now, they had plenty of challenges, too. Yes, siree. I am grateful for my growth.

January 24, 1998

What a wonderful "to a bright future" surprise party Tom had for Me! How excited I was to see everyone there to congratulate me on the end of my long treatment, and share my hope and faith for remission. I still can't believe Tom was able to keep everything hushed! He made a lot of phone calls whenever I was in the shower. Lucky for everyone I take mine at night since we have to get up at 5:00 A.M. for work these days. Amazingly, he spread the word about a top secret gathering and pulled off a grand affair. He added lots of special touches: flowers, a rainbow cake, colorful balloons, and rainbow decorations. I don't believe he forgot a single thing; it gave such a tug on my heart. I'm a bit silly—perhaps corny—but I thought it was wonderful! These are the little things that are so special in my life. And what an eloquent speech he gave to me and our guests!

Tom is not a man of many words, especially in a crowd. As his voice quivered and his eyes filled with tears, I looked around the room and saw warmth and sincerity in all the faces. I'm certain they were thinking much as I, what a wonderful husband, what a great guy! His message was truly heartfelt by all! He sure fits the description of the song, *Baby You're the Best* by Carlie Simon.

I sit here thinking of when Tom and I first dated, I told Mom that this new boyfriend of mine was somewhat quiet, and maybe he was

Barbara Dooling

even a bit short for me. How critical we women can be when in search of Mister Right. But Mom reminded me that I should give him time. She added that Dad, who is also quite short, seemed to be ten feet tall to her sometimes. Mom was right. She has so much wisdom. Well, Tom has sprouted many feet since I married him! How immensely fortunate I am. I surely appreciate this man I married.

My "Bright Future, Stay Well" party lifted my spirits. The decoration were so appropriate. A bright yellow sunbrightened the rainbow cake; "To a bright future" was scrawled across the top. Oh Tom, I love you, my darling!

There were two special guest appearances! Somehow Tom found the phone numbers of my new friends Ann and Linda. I was especially overwhelmed to see them because our correspondence has been mostly by phone or through greeting cards. Unfortunately, we do share the same diagnosis of breast cancer, but these lovely ladies are survivors and have inspired me with their own stories of strength and courage. Linda hasn't forgotten me and took the time to attend my party, and Ann traveled from Rhode Island to share the day, too.

Now it's my turn to thank everyone...

To Tom, Best Husband Award

I love you for putting joy into each hour, making me laugh when I wanted to cry. Each and every day since my treatment began, you kept my worn out body fueled by your love and strength, restoring and healing my soul. You never feared that I might lose my breast. You said, "Do whatever it takes to be rid of the cancer." I needed to hear that I would still be attractive to you. You never cared that I'd lose my hair. I could have chosen a milder form

Impossible Choices

of chemotherapy which would have saved my pretty curls. But you said, "Kill the damned cancer!" I loved how you asked to rub my shiny head and then tickled it with gentle kisses. You told me how pretty my head was. You said that you loved my head. I love you for saying that!

Thank you for clutching me tightly and kissing me good night. Since the day we were married, we still say "I love you" every night. May the honeymoon last forever. I love you!

To Mom and Dad, Best Parents Award

You must have been devastated to learn of my diagnosis, but you never showed more enormous strength, faith, and courage. You convinced me to have courage. I had to beg God for that because I didn't seem to have much. Thank you for your love and support which you have given me throughout my entire life.

Mom, I'm aware of your daily prayers, and that you and Dad say the rosary for me. You are my ticket into heaven. You and Dad have taught me about strong family bonds, the true value of life, and love of animals and nature. You encouraged me to smell the flowers, feel the sunshine on my face, respect the rain, and to look for the rainbow. You directed me to seek solace and answers from the ocean. You told me to yell as loud as I can to the mountains and that they would talk back, giving me reason and answers. You instilled daily the message to love myself, to be committed to relationships such as friendships and marriage. You always said that giving is rewarding. How do I ever thank you for all this? It is quite special and so are you.

The most important gift of life is knowing how much I am loved. This sees me through the darkest hours when I feel frightened and helpless. I am so grateful to my wonderful,

Barbara Dooling

wonderful parents. I remember so well how Mom sang sweet lullabies, and how she would rock me and hold me tightly as she twirled her fingers around my hair. I still dream thoughts of my childhood and her nurturing ways. And to Dad, I will always be your little girl. Your bunny, your princess who danced upon your toes. I love you both!

To Russ and Ann, (Annabelle)

Russ, I know… I know you used to change my diapers. How can I ever thank you for that? Washed my mouth out with soap for saying a naughty word. I don't swear anymore (well, hardly ever). You never could make a camper out of me, could you? I still can't pitch a tent. Hey, where's the blowup furniture? You mean tents don't come with carpets? Don't like mosquitoes. Don't like bugs. Give me the Hilton with cable and rugs. You want me to fit all my "stuff" into a duffel bag? But I like my suitcase! What? I can't bring my blow-dryer? I didn't think I was going to like that trip, but I did! How corny, we even sang songs around the campfire.

Moving on to later years—thanks for consoling me after the break up with my first love. How right you were to tell me I'd find love again. Better than before, right? THAT'S FOR SURE!! Thanks for taping my wedding poem to Tom for the "imperial affair," sure took us a long time to get the recording right. Lots of laughter and tears that day. Thank you for your love and support. I love you.

To Ann,

Ann, thanks for the meals on wheels during my treatment. Free delivery. Mmmmmm good! Soup to nuts! Thank you for always taking such wonderful care of me, even when I was little. I don't like mustard and cheese sandwiches anymore! I still have the cats from the Disney movie *Aristocrats*. We saw that in the seventies in Connecticut, remember? I love you.

To Ken,

You couldn't attend my Stay-well surprise party, but thanks for the telephone call to say you were thinking of me. You are always thinking of me. You're the John-boy Walton of our family. Oh how I loved those songs you played on your guitar for me when I was little. How was it they all had my name in them? Kind and gentle. Loving and sincere. You always made me feel special. Still do. You made the best Christmas out of "the Christmas that almost wasn't." Dad was in the hospital and we still hadn't gotten our tree. Surprised us on Christmas Eve with the greatest, fattest tree! All the presents were decorated with reindeer and Santa's. We strung popcorn and cranberries for the first time. It was even a white Christmas to top it off. I'll never forget it. How I always missed you when you left! It was sad saying good-bye. Then I grew up and got the key to your house in Newport. Party at Kenny's... All the time, anytime, black tie parties till four o'clock in the morning. No lines. No waiting. Step right up. I'm Kenny's sister, Barbara. We never had to pay the cover charge at the clubs either. Beaches, yachts, and parties. What a life! Remember your wealthy friend asking, "What kind of a boat do you have, Barbara?" I answered, "Aaaahhhhhmmmm. I don't have a boat, but I have a car." Did he really think I had a boat? Ah, well... I still don't have one. Tee hee. Did I forget to mention the concerts at the park near the ocean? How about the time my friends and I rented a room in a mansion? Were we out of control or what? Can't say I never sowed my oats. Thank you for my big surprise on my wedding day. Did you have to make me cry though? Grateful for all your phone calls through my treatments and for your love and support. I love you!

To Paul and Maureen,

Paul, I miss you. Even though you live in Colorado, you always sent cards and prayers during my illness. Paul… "Pauli Wogg" remember my little nicknames? How could you forget? You never minded, or did you? Sorry. My taxi service. How could you even think of moving to Colorado? Never made me get rid of my cats even though you had asthma. Oops! You mean you couldn't breathe? Thanks for funding my trip to Florida in 1979. Lots of fun on all my trips thereafter, especially to Colorado. The best was when our whole family went out to see your wedding. What a splendid time we had, but how funny you were. The first day, you tried that itinerary on us. We wanted no part of sticking to a schedule on our vacation. The ski trip was excellent. Vail, Colorado in a snow storm. What fluffy snow! You took quite a spill. The abominable snowman. Ha ha ha! You're too much. Sure do miss you. Maybe I'm due for another Colorado adventure. Maureen, thanks for your sincere words of encouragement. You've been so good to my brother. I'm glad he has you. I love you both!

To Mary and Eddie,

Mary, best hostess. Best parties. Best barbecues. Best house. Best cook. Best laundry service. Best baby-sitter. Best friend. Thank heaven for sisters. Thank heaven for my sister. My savior. My only sister. I treasure you! Fancy food for my surprise stay well party. Always the wind beneath my wings. Stayed with us after my surgery and during my first chemotherapy treatments. Daily calls. How will I ever thank you? You are always taking care of me. Even since I was a little girl. You thought Mom and Dad had me just for you. I was

Impossible Choices

your little cuddle doll. You played dress up with me instead of with your own dolls. Dropped me a lot. Stole me out of my own bed to sleep with you at night. Broke the news to me about Santa Claus. But there really is a Santa Claus and I married him! You never kept me from tagging along. Won't ever forget your surprise visit to Boston to deliver flowers for my birthday. I know how you hate to drive in Boston. Let me be an assistant coach when your daughter, Alicia was born—Yikes! That was scary but I remained calm, cool, and mostly collected. Helped with my wedding plans. Thank you for all the extra things you did that added to my special day. And… for always making me feel special. Thank you for all your love and support. *Eddie, Eddie, he's my man, if he can't fix it, no one can!* Tall and lean, but never mean. What a guy! What a guy! What a guy! I love you both!

To Geno and Karen,

Were unable to attend my Surprise Stay-well party, but haven't missed much else in my life. Thank you for the prayer for the ill card. Never knew they had that kind. I always thought mass cards were for the deceased. Whew! Geno, did I ever thank you for the "live killer bee" you left for me when I was little? Well I really must. It was so thoughtful of you, knowing how much I disliked insects! The plastic container was labeled: *Caution, live killer bee inside.* You left it right on my night stand. There was a real bee in it!

My confidant in high school. Double dated at the prom. Told my boyfriends you would shoot them with Dad's gun if they got out of line… even though dad never had a gun. Took me to parties. Made sure I listened to cool music—*Pin Ball Wizard.* White horse beach wearing green trash bags during a hurricane. Bob Seger. Miniature golf. Concerts. Where did all those carefree days go? I loved them. I

Barbara Dooling

love you. By the way, I wasn't adopted. Mom and Dad didn't find me. And I don't have baggy underwear (anymore). Oh yeah, if you ever see "Apple Annie" tell her I was asking for her.

Karen, thanks for writing endless cards and letters to me when I lived in California. You'll never know how much I looked forward to them. I was so homesick. I remember Geno sent me a Winnie The Pooh teddy to keep me company. I was so touched that he remembered how I loved pooh bear. I love you both!

To Mom and Dad Dooling,

Best meals. Best roast beast. Most wonderful in-laws a girl could have. Made food for the party celebration. Have the finest daycare in town. Opens at six o'clock in the morning. Never closes. Sometimes does overnights. No paid holidays, sick days, overtime anytime. You ought to quit that crummy job. How do I ever thank you? Always there to help with our Kara, especially during my treatments. Grampy is kind, warm, and honest. Wonder where Tom gets it from? Grammy, alike can do most anything and is always ready with a joke. Shares her things, especially her special china tea cup. Thinking back, you folks saved Tom and I from the Pine Street Inn when our apartment house got sold. Thanks for taking us in until we bought our own home. Helped renovate our new home. Grampy did the worst room—better known as Grumpy's dungeon. Best vacation cottage in Maine. Rent's real cheap at zero dollars per week. Really should raise the price. Awfully glad you don't. Always seem to have a "get out of jail" free card. Oops, I mean "get out of a jam" free card. Don't ever change your phone number. Thank you for your love and support. I love you both!

Impossible Choices

To Margaret and Jimmy,

Marg, you always know what to say… so genuine, funny, and always helpful. Jimmy is so kind and big hearted, that's why we chose him to be Kara's Godfather. Not only big-hearted, he's big—really big. Poor Kara screams at the sight of him… poor Jimmy. I love you both!

To Tricia and Bill,

Tricia, you are warm, friendly and easy to talk with. What a beautiful person inside and out! You and I like a lot of the same things: artists, Victorian décor, clothing styles and more. Huh! We both had a horse and carriage on our wedding day. I always feel comfortable and welcome in your home. Bill's hearty, jovial laugh is amusing! I love you both!

To Carolyn and Paul,

Best house. Best people. Best parties. Best music! Thanks Paul for telling me you like short hair on women, it made me feel grrrreat when I took my wig off to show my new growth. I love you!

To Donna and Jeff,

Donna, you are full of life, free-spirited, giving—most beautiful blue eyes I ever saw. Jeff is true to his word, individual, generous—what a great couple! I love you both!

February 12, 1998

I have joined a breast cancer support group! I want to learn more about the disease by educating myself and finding new resources. Now that the treatment is over, I am afraid because I'm not actively doing anything to fight the cancer. I feel like I'm in limbo. What protects me now from the cancer? How do I keep it from returning? How do I deal with the fear that every ache or pain is the cancer? I'll continue to alternate between seeing my oncologist and surgeon every three months, but I'm still scared! When I was in treatment, I was constantly being watched. It's a weird feeling not to be killing the cancer off anymore. I'm glad to be done with chemo and radiation... happy that my time is my own again... but I feel kind of all alone. Lost. I really need to seek new ways to remain a survivor!

So the support group will be great! I'm a little afraid because I can't help wondering if I bond with these women, what will happen if one dies? It will be good to chat with women who are experiencing many of the same feelings and fears, but I don't want to hear any bad stuff. No, I don't want to listen to stories about cancer recurrence. I guess I will give it a chance and see how it goes.

April 22, 1998

Happy birthday to me, happy birthday to me, happy birthday to, Mommy Barbara, happy birthday to me! Another birthday! I love it. Thirty-seven! I'm grateful to have this day! Tom and darling Kara Elizabeth made a lopsided cake for me. The chocolate frosting was all over the counter and Kara's face. Her clothes and hair wore it too. What a ragamuffin! My two favorite people in this whole world helped me blow out all my candles. Kara was so funny. She wanted to keep lighting the flames and puff them out over and over again. We did just that. Then we ate cake!

May 8, 1998

Spring! Daffodils! Lily's! Easter! It was just January when my

Impossible Choices

treatment ended and already my hair is growing back. It's still very short, but I do have hair! Wonderful, downy soft wisps and fine bangs! I have a brown head! Feels awesome, and no gray! I wondered about that! Didn't really care if it came back gray or purple—just wanted stubble. I've got more than that! It's me again when I look into the mirror. No more wig… no more turbans and hats… no more baldness. Imagine, all that time without hair. It's me!

May 10, 1998

I feel so wonderful on this, my second Mother's Day! Thank you God! I'm still here!

May 24, 1998

Pushed my sweet child in her carriage all the way to the park. A mile uphill. I huffed and I puffed; I'm out of shape between the surgery and chemo. The yards we passed were trimmed with new spring grass, and budding flowers and trees. I welcomed the cool breeze against my sweaty skin. The playground was crowded with mothers, fathers, and squealing children. There were so many pregnant women and new born babies around. It's hard to think about the future. I should just be so lucky to be here with Kara, but I can't help wanting to have another baby.

Kara popped the buckle and squirmed out through the bottom of the carriage. She is too funny! The minute she hit the ground, she was off and running every which way. I am truly amazed at how fast and strong she is! She's only eighteen months, yet she tries to climb the big jungle gym. Whenever I try to help her, she shouts, "I do it! I do it!" She ran me ragged and surely tuckered herself out too. I can't get the cancer out of my mind today. Spending time with Kara at the park breaks my heart these days. I try to stay focused and positive about my prognosis, but the cancer bummers always leak into my thoughts. Kara is such a beautiful, high spirited child. What will happen to her if I should die? She needs me! And I don't want to be deprived of watching her grow up! I've got to get rid of these unspeakable thoughts. No more writing about such nonsense!

July 20, 1998

Our summer vacation's here at last! We're up at the cottage in Old Orchard Beach. Here for two weeks… I packed for ten! Well, ya know how chilly it gets at night on the beach. Must have plenty of clothes for Kara. The first few days we spent lounging in the warm sun. Kara was content all day chasing waves and building sand castles. She loves to crush her peaks and splash in her moats. Daddy gets annoyed because he does most of the work and Kara wrecks it within seconds. Those tiny feet demolish his prideful sand sculptures. I have to remind him that Kara is a toddler and he's the grown up! We take lazy strolls along the shoreline looking for crabs and shells. After we eat our picnic lunch, we snooze if Kara permits it! The trick is to run her like a puppy all over the beach… get her real tired… and maybe, just maybe she naps. I wish I could bottle some of her energy!

July 23, 1998

Went downtown tonight. Kara had a ball going on all the kiddy rides. She absolutely loves the motorcycles! Daddy is excited to have a biker chick at long last! Mommy doesn't really like his Harley. After we took a hundred pictures of Kara gloating at the amusement park, we licked soft serve ice cream at the pier. Kara ran up and down the length of the wharf without ever stopping for a breath. Those little legs don't ever want to stop running, running,

Impossible Choices

running. She might have escaped us if it weren't for crashing into the crowds of people. I love how she looks over her shoulder to see if we're watching her. Then she takes off full speed, laughing because she thinks that she's getting away with something. What a doll! I could eat her up!

July 25, 1998

Kara gets up at the crack of dawn—literally. We keep reminding her that we're on vacation, but she is so used to getting up at five o'clock in the morning because Tom and I both work. So, we've been taking turns getting up with her. Tom is great. He takes her out in the stroller and walks to Ocean Park. Along his way, he picks flowers for me... some wild... some he steals out of front yards! I have quite the collection—two bouquets, in fact. They really spruce up the cottage. In the kitchen, I have black-eyed Susan's, white daisies, purple wisteria, and some green fern. The living room displays wild roses, bright yellow dahlias, branching yellow clusters of goldenrod, delicate white lily of the valley, large pink lilies, orange tiger lilies, and some I haven't a clue what they are! I declare! He adds a different species everyday! Kara gets to present them to me. She tiptoes into the cottage with her face and little body practically hidden behind these florid clusters. Oh my, I just love my life... my little family. God, please keep me well!

September 2, 1998

On this crisp day with the weather soon giving way to autumn, a young mother of two little girls lay in a hospital bed, losing her battle with breast cancer. Our paths crossed only because we share the same dreadful disease. I was asked by my support group facilitator to visit this ailing woman; she is close to my age. Thinking that

Barbara Dooling

perhaps it would help her to talk with another "bosom buddy," I visited Annmarie this afternoon. Not knowing what to say, I was reluctant to enter her hospital room.

I wondered how I would even introduce myself, and if she would want this stranger to be with her when she was so ill. I had little information about Annmarie, mainly that we both had small children and we both had breast cancer. I'm fourteen months out from my original diagnosis and doing well with no signs of cancer recurrence. She's fifteen months out from her original diagnosis and dying. Even as I write this, I have chills up my spine.

The cancer has rapidly spread to her liver and all treatment is failing. I was terrified to meet her because I kept thinking this could be me. I wondered what in the world was I going to say to this person to make a difference.

I entered this typical hospital room, which was filled with flowers situated all about the window sill and on top of the heater. There were green leafed plants, budding floral plants, and fresh cut flowers in makeshift vases. Hard candies were scattered on the night stand along with tissues and magazines that appeared unread. There in the bed, as pale as the sheets, my new friend Annmarie lay sleeping. As I looked at her, I wondered how long I was going to know her… I was aware that these are the final days of her life.

I backtracked toward the door trying to slip out of the room without disturbing her rest. As if sensing my presence, she opened her eyes. The sweetest voice asked, "Do I know you? Please come in." I introduced myself just as I had rehearsed moments before. I told her about my treatment for the breast cancer. After that, all I could think to say was that I would pray for her and her children. I walked to Annmarie's bedside, taking her hand firmly into my own. I leaned over and kissed her forehead. She asked me to stay a while,

Impossible Choices

though she drifted back into a doze. I did stay, sitting quietly for thirty minutes. I was feeling just awful. I left her without speaking again, and I returned to my own home and family.

September 5, 1998

I continue my half-hour visits daily, sometimes twice a day. I always leave Annmarie alone with her family or other visitors; I don't want to impose on her time with them. I have recently witnessed Sheila's mother die. Painful as that was, somehow it was easier to accept because she was much older than Annmarie. The death of a loved-one is always sad, but none as mournful as when someone is robbed of their youth. When death comes early we feel cheated. Though I can clearly see that Annmarie is a beautiful woman, the disease ravishing her body has taken its toll. Her skin is almost transparent, her lips so chapped that they bleed, and her stomach is swollen with an enlarged liver and fluid. Sometimes I hand her a warmed face cloth so she can cleanse herself. She uses the hospital's makeshift mouth refreshers. These are mint flavored pink foam balls on a stick which I assume take the place of a toothbrush. Whenever her lips bleed, I give her some ice chips to keep her mouth moist. I don't think too much about this new nursing position. I just keep visiting. I'm compelled to keep going, determined to help her in some way.

Today we chatted about everything and nothing. I finally conjured up the courage to ask her if she wanted me to do some writing for her. My hope is to write a letter from her to each of her daughters since she's too weak to do it herself. At first she didn't want any part of my idea. She fears it will be like writing a good-bye letter to her children. She says by doing this, she will be giving up. I explained that I've been writing journals for Kara even before

Barbara Dooling

I got cancer. It's my way of talking to my little one—heart-to-heart. I write my present feelings so I won't forget them even though my baby is too young to understand. Plus writing my feelings down helps to soothe me. Annmarie agreed that she wanted to do this for her own daughters, April and Rachel. Thus, today we started with pen and paper! Annmarie talked while I penned.

September 12, 1998

I've finished gathering information about her two daughters, and last night I stayed up until the early hours of the morning, writing frantically and piecing together my scribbled notes. Annmarie has become much weaker and I fear that she will not live to give her letters to those girls. I returned to the hospital very early this morning. Thank God she's still alive! At seven o'clock in the morning, I read them aloud. We laughed and we cried; what good friends we have become. Then I came home to write another letter. I've decided to put it in my journal—the home of all my deepest emotions.

To my new friend, Annmarie,

Though I have only known you just two weeks, you have touched my heart so thoroughly. It is easy to see that you have marked the lives of many. It is unfortunate that we met under these circumstances, and not for a happier reason.

Giving much thought to what you shared with me about yourself, I have come to realize that people face their destinies in many different ways. You said prisoners of war and early pioneers faced death everyday. You asked me how some people survived and others perished. I could only answer with survival of the fittest. You continued by saying that the survivors never gave up hope. What

Impossible Choices

tremendous strength and courage you have—and have given to me. How could you fail with the love you receive from your devoted husband at your side? You have the support of your wonderful mother and the affection of your siblings. I see how your own children, two beautiful daughters, light up your eyes and inspire your every breath. All this I witness and it touches me.

I continue to visit you daily even though my heart is heavy. I asked myself, why this woman tugs at me so. I know the answer. You are genuine; how fortunate I am to have the opportunity to get to know you. It was fun swapping stories about our husbands and how we met them. You proudly shared how you married the letter carrier of your employer. You began to reminisce, declaring, "David delivered a valentine to me and asked me out on a date. I think he liked my long red hair. I have loved him ever since."

I peeked at your head that now reveals fuzzy new hair growth. You'd lost your mane of red during chemotherapy treatment. I wondered what you looked like before this. We talked and laughed about our love life like two young school girls. I'm so glad that I asked you if you wanted me to jot down some of our conversations. I felt that you really wanted to but had been unable to bring yourself to get started. How often you became too tired and weak, and you drifted off to sleep during our chats. But you were always smiling. You must have been dreaming of a mailman and a very special Valentine.

As your health continued to deteriorate, your breathing was labored and you could barely sit up. But one morning, I was astonished when I stepped into your room. You greeted me with such warmth as you said, "Let's talk about my two little girls." I couldn't believe how you perked up. Your eyes opened wider than I had seen them all week. Propping yourself up in the bed, you

Barbara Dooling

began chatting away. Your energy level was terrific! With joy in your heart and a twinkle in your eyes, you told me all about your precious lambs. I was trying to take notes, and I could hardly keep up with you.

Think about those sweet darlings, Annmarie, when you are frightened or sad and they will surely lift your spirit. You are such a lovely person, truly a fine woman. I'd like to know you forever and I shall do so in my heart.

With much affection, your new friend, *Barbara Dooling*

September 14, 1998

I am heartbroken that Annmarie will never read that letter. I'm devastated today. She has succumbed to breast cancer. She died in her own home with her family at her side. I am glad that her husband David took her out of the hospital to be at home. I cannot write any more… I do not know what to say. I think that I just need to go have a good cry.

September 17, 1998

It took a magnitude of energy for me to attend her wake, but I went. Again, I saw my own husband, my own little girl, and myself in their place. But I thought to myself, you're stronger than you know.

October 4, 1998

What a beautiful sunny October morning! Along with thousands of other people, I walked the nearly six mile *Making Strides Against Breast Cancer* around Boston's Charles River. The walk was emotionally challenging for me. The most difficult part was seeing all those people who walked in memory of someone

Impossible Choices

they had loved and lost to this devastating disease.

Although there is a tremendous need for money in research to improve treatments, better yet to find a cure, I chose to donate my sponsors' contributions to Annmarie's two children. That's right! I collected money by reaching out to every person I know, using my old wedding list of family, friends, and coworkers. Amazingly, my sponsors and I raised over twelve hundred dollars. Together, we made a difference in someone else's life. What a terrific opportunity to make "stone soup."

It was more like minestrone! Ha, ha, ha. I surely remember the classic story about stone soup. Everyone in the town gives something to make the soup. Someone gives the pot. Several others give the vegetables. And lastly, some help with the seasoning. Together, a delicious soup is made for all to share!

October 15, 1998

It's late on a Saturday afternoon. Just got back from delivering the donation to Annmarie's husband David. What a day! Their two little girls April and Rachel eagerly came to the door to greet me. April, who is four years old, has chestnut hair and dark brown eyes. Rachel is two and she has the most beautiful, thick blond hair. Rachel was a little shy and was hiding behind her daddy. I instantly fell in love with this family.

The girls were bare foot and their hair hung freely without barrettes or bows. I introduced myself to them as their mommy's good friend. I told the girls how much their mommy had talked about them and how much she loved them. I received an instant smile from the two of them. I was deeply touched by their innocence.

David showed me some family photographs. Annmarie really was so beautiful and her auburn hair was incredibly lovely. As I

Barbara Dooling

looked at those pictures, I couldn't help thinking back to when I met Annmarie... she was nearly bald and so sickly. It was hard to imagine I was looking at the same person. There was an elegant wedding picture of Annmarie and David hanging in the living room. The whole house was cheerful and filled with happy memories. Yah, that whole place shouted Annmarie; her hand-crafted wreaths and artwork decorated the entire house. Everywhere I looked, there was a woman's touch. I felt Annmarie's presence and I missed her. I could only wonder about this family's grief.

But the children were excited to have company. They were happy and playful. I asked David how everyone was coping. He was positive in his response. He told me they would all muddle through somehow. That they would stick together and help each other and that they would manage. David is a good person and he loves his two little girls very much. It shows. I'm proud of this man. He is determined to keep his family together and make a life for them. He talks about their future and he has a plan. I know he and the girls are truly going to make it. April and Rachel tragically lost their mother, but they are not going to lose their father, too. David will see to it that those children have a happy life.

When it was time for me to leave, we all said good-bye. Again the girls were jumping and restless with excitement. It was a pleasant visit. I told David and the girls that I would be sure to keep in touch. April and Rachel are eager to meet Kara. Kara is just two years old and now she will have two wonderful new friends. My girlie-girl is full of spunk like Rachel. They will all have lots of fun together.

November 26, 1998

Thanksgiving Day! So much to be thankful for. We had dinner at

Impossible Choices

Mom and Dad's house; everyone made it this year. There was Kenny and his two kids, Mary and her family, Geno and his clan, Tom and I with Little Miss Kara. Dad said a tear jerker prayer. He thanked God that I am still here! All of our lives are one big acknowledgment; we should all be happy to be here. You just never know what tomorrow will bring. After dinner we called Paul and Maureen in Colorado, and Russ and Ann came later for desert. Christmas will be here before we know it and we'll spend that day with Tom's family.

Family. I'm so glad to have family! Can't help thinking that I'd love to give Kara a brother or sister. It's too soon to tell if we can even think about another pregnancy. I must be thankful for today—for all the many things that I have today.

December 12, 1998

I'm sneaking in an entry from Kara... in her own words, using her voice. This is how she sounds:

Hello from Kara Elizabeth Dooling, and Happy Holidays

That's "Helloooo from Kara Lizabeeet Duuulin!" I'm two years old and it's Christmastime. Mommy and Daddy say hi, too. They are busy decorating the house for Christmas, so I will tell you all about the latest happenings with me...

I offered to help them with all the trimming festivities, but mommy didn't like the way I crushed all the caroling dolls. I was only trying to pull their hair out to see if it was real. Daddy wouldn't let me help with the window candle lights either. Those glass bulbs are shiny enough to eat! Well I did help with the tree until it was time for a wee little nap.

When I woke up, the tree was awwwwll done like magic and it was beautiful. I was so excited! I kept saying, "Prrreeeety, prrreeeety

Barbara Dooling

and I luv it, I luv it!" Each time I walk by our tree, I kiss the ornaments on the lower branches. There is Winnie The Pooh, of course; Tigger, Rabbit, and Roo, and some kind of horse that rocks. I also have a very funny Santa and some little jingle bells. I like to ping the bells and laugh. A bit higher on the tree are the ornaments that mommy calls, "Verrrry pecial." I am not allowed to touch these at all. It's okay because I really like my pooh bear and friends. I think our whole tree is verrrry verrrry pecial.

What a great birthday party I had in November... that's "ovember" with my cousins and friends. Everything was decorated with Noah's Ark for two. Mommy set up a table and put a whole bunch of toy animals all around an ark. There were two of each kind. We gave each child at my party a chance to pick two each of those animals. A real petting zoo came to my house with baby goats, a pig, sheep, tiny chicks, rabbits, a huge snake, and an iguana. I was not afraid and petted every one of them. The baby chicks and soft fluffy rabbits made me laugh when I held them. I tried not to squish them. Later, we had animal face painting. It seemed that all the children except for me were in some sort of animal disguise. I would not sit in a chair long enough for this creative game. When it came time to blow out my candles, I knew just what to do. Before the birthday song was over, I gave a big puff and out went the flames! I sang along with everyone, *"Happy day tuuuuy, happy day tuuuuy."* I laughed and clapped, and mommy cried. When mommy and daddy eat by candlelight, I sing the birthday song and try to blow out their candles.

Now that I am two years old, I am getting sooooo big—well, not exactly. I am quite petite, just like my mommy. Daddy says I have the cutest little buns. He tells mommy that too. I have the most delicate features, but I am far from fragile. My daddy plays rough and tough

Impossible Choices

with me. I do not like to wear ribbons or bows in my hair. Every time mommy tries that stuff, I pull them right out. Mommy says, "pretty Kara." And I say, "no prreeeety, no prreeeety."

I am talking a lot more and repeat even the big words. I can say: I have it, Kara have it, I luv it, I luv you, bless you mommy, bless you daddy (after they sneeze or cough,) excuse me, I poop, Daddy poops, read story, I get out crib Mommy, I go shop'n Mommy, my book, my dollar, Daddy's money, and soooo much more. I like to call my nana on the telephone and say, "Helloooo, Nana. I luv me, Nana." (That's I love you, Nana.) I say "Yes peeeez and no tank you." Sometimes I like to go out in the rain. I holler, "Outside, mommy." And mommy tells me it's raining, Kara. I shout, "My coat. Outside, Mommy. Rain, rain, rain." My alphabet is coming along very well; "abcdfglmpuv... won't you sing me." I sing, "Twinkle twinkle little star up above were sky are." I count, "One, two, three, four, eight, nine, eleven." I am doing much better with my colors, too. For a while, I called everything blue. Daddy would point to a red balloon and I would proudly say, "Blue, Daddy."

Each night my mommy or daddy reads to me on their big bed. I can turn the pages two at a time. Sometimes I jump on the big bed, and Mommy yells, "No more monkeys jumping on the bed!" I like to stand up because I can see lots of fine things on Mommy's bureau. She lets me wind up the beautiful glass music boxes. There is beauty and the beast, Peter Rabbit, and a mommy mouse named Hunca Munca, rocking her baby Mice in a crib. Daddy gets nervous that I will break them. Mommy just tells me that magic word, "special." I repeat, "pecial, very pecial." She lets me hold the glass pieces on the big bed. Mommy says special people will have special things. She says I am a special people.

I have been learning to share. It is a very difficult thing, this sharing business. I like the words, I, me, and mine. I don't like the words, him and her. Although, it is much nicer to have someone to play with. Mommy takes me to a play group on her days off from work. We also like to visit the library. Now that I can read picture books, I like to pull them all off the shelves. The library is a very fun place to be. I push the swinging door that leads to the "lady." Mommy calls her the librarian, and I call her "lady." Whenever I am at the library, I do try to use my indoor voice or whisper like I'm telling a secret. That lady makes sure I talk softly and put all the books back on the shelf. I like her.

When we don't visit the library, mommy takes me to the park. Wow! I run, jump, and climb on everything. My favorite is the motorcycle. Seems to be Daddy's favorite, too. Whenever we have a family day at the park, Daddy sits on the little motorcycle and revs it up. Mommy tells him to get off, but he never does. My daddy has a real motorcycle called a Harley Davidson. It is very loud.

Most importantly, I am quite interested in the potty chair. Mommy and Daddy think this is the greatest thing. My dolly does too. I am not afraid to sit on the big potty even though I'm so little. I don't fear too many things, not even the time-out chair. Sometimes I sit in this time-out chair more than the potty chair. I am very independent, tenacious, and strong. At least those are the words I hear mommy use when she talks to my pediatrician. My doctor can't believe my strength for such a little girl. Mommy says I have spirit and spunk for a tiny person! Yep, that's me, little Miss Kara Elizabeth Dooling, that's "Kara Lizabeeet Duuulin."

Mommy has a new shelf with a wonderful collection of angels displayed on it. Can you believe I'm there, too? My picture is right there next to all the cherubs. Mommy says I am her angel, sent to her right from God. Wow! Daddy says that mommy and I are his

Impossible Choices

angels. We will make snow angels this winter when it snows. We believe in all angels, don't you? May your angels keep you happy and safe all the year through.

January 8, 1999

I'm back! Isn't Kara a sweetie? This last year before the new millennium has indeed started with a bang. What's happening is astonishing. I'm flabbergasted! I'm dumbfounded! Today has been interlaced with loops and knots. I don't know where to begin. I'm one and half years out from the diagnosis and I've had no symptoms of recurrence. I've been feeling pretty good. My days are filled with happiness and gratitude because I am still here on this earth with my family. I'm trying to put the whole cancer ordeal behind me, although that often takes tremendous effort. I have a little procedure: I convince my mind that the cancer is completely gone. Sometimes I feel much like a hypochondriac, thinking every ache or pain in my body is a cancer rebound. Funny how often I discover I have cancer each month—at least four times a week. But each time, I've done very well at fighting these fears with all my might. And so on this eighth day of January 1999, when I went to see my surgeon for a routine follow-up, I did not think cancer. I thought future.

Once again, I had a list of questions about getting pregnant. The list, like one for Santa, is constantly on my mind. The tally is there the whole year through. I'm constantly thinking about it, and I'm always trying to be good so that I can have everything on the list. I've played by all the rules being very cautious not to become pregnant until I'm two years cancer free from the date of my diagnosis. That's what my oncologist has recommended.

On this cold January day, a snowstorm was about to fall on

Barbara Dooling

Boston and on me too. My appointment began in the usual way, waiting endlessly for the doctor. She's well worth the wait—a highly regarded breast surgeon among her colleagues. I too, respect her and find her to be a superb physician. I have learned to utilize the waiting room time and always carry my journal with me. Alas, my name was called. I was brought into the examining room. Before I knew it, as if a wind came through the window and blew the list from my hands, I never got to ask my questions. The doctor had an ashen look on her face. It was a gray face that usually belonged to me, not her. A mere mention of some lower back pain resulted in great concern from her. I thought to myself, but I always have back strain because I work on a computer a lot.

The doctor pulled a report from my chart, excused herself from the room, and closed the door behind her. I heard a lot of voices and I began to sweat. What in heaven was going on? My doctor returned with some curious and very disturbing news. Based on a previous bone scan that I had six months prior to this visit, it appeared that the cancer had quite possibly metastasized to my bones. Wait just a minute. Let me think. Let me absorb this. No, it couldn't be. Six months prior, I was told the result was normal. I asked, "How could it be? Why have six months passed with no indication about this?" She expressed that perhaps I was thinking of my mammogram which was done a month later than the scan. No, I am not mistaken. I was told the bone scan was normal. I asked the doctor why this bone scan was not questioned originally if there was a mention of metastasis. If there was cancer present what of it now… a whole six months later?

She did not answer the question but went on to explain about bone metastasis. I listened intently as she told me there is no cure. No cure? Surely I was going to pass out. It couldn't be true… not

Impossible Choices

again… no, not again. I beg you, God, no. I was clutching my crucifix that I wear everyday on a delicate gold chain around my neck. She continued telling me they could try to treat the cancer like a chronic illness, and keep it at bay for as long as possible. She said they had a lot of tricks up their sleeves. At the end of the conversation, she told me I would need to complete a series of tests in order to be sure the cancer was not anywhere else. She asked if I wanted her to call my husband. My heart was racing much the same way as the first day I was diagnosed. I was thinking, my God, what am I going to do? What ever am I going to do?

I phoned Tom from the surgeon's office. I wanted to tell him the news myself. My gemstone, my rock assured me that I would be fine. He counseled, "Don't panic. You don't know for sure. No one knows for sure." I remained at the hospital for blood work and a chest and abdominal CT scan to rule out any spread of cancer to soft tissue such as the lungs or liver. A repeat bone scan was ordered for the following Tuesday. This would show if cancer has, in fact, spread to the bone as it appears in the previous scan from six months ago.

Nine hours later, I left the hospital. My car was covered in snow. My gosh! I had forgotten about the predicted storm. It was now rush hour in downtown Boston and snowing very hard. I removed the heavy wet snow from the windshield to uncover a surprise from the meter maid. I laughed. How trivial. Over an hour later I arrived home safely. At least the snow kept me from thinking about what I would have otherwise been thinking of, which surely would have gotten me in a wreck. My beautiful family, who was safe and warm inside, gave me the grandest welcome home. It was indeed grand to be home. But as tired and worn out as I felt, I was driven by some force to sort photographs and get them into albums. At two o'clock in the morning, Tom insisted I stop the nonsense, and I finally went to bed, but never to sleep.

January 9, 1999

Now I have the weekend to be haunted by my worst fears. Tom's done his best to keep my thoughts off the cancer. I'm doing my best not to cry, especially in front of Kara. I don't want to frighten her. Inevitably, she did catch me sobbing today, and the wee little lamb put her tiny arm around my neck and whispered, "Mommy, you feel better. I make you feel better." Her small but strong hand patted my back and she gave me a healing kiss like the ones she gives to her dollies. This child of mine is quite special. She is truly special, and I am so lucky to have her in my life.

January 10, 1999

Last night, Saturday evening, though I was immensely tired, I lay in bed staring into the darkness. I've been so anxious. Tears streamed off my cheeks and onto my pillow. I tried to be silent so that I wouldn't wake Tom. Well, at least *he* is sleeping I thought. But he wasn't—not at all. He reached for my hand underneath the blanket. My icy, negative thoughts melted as if warmed by his tight grip. The heat of his love and concern went directly into my hand spreading right through my body. I imagined it rushing into my blood and throughout my anatomy, and curing me. Can good lovin' and affection get rid of cancer? It did tonight.

Today, I'm back at the dining room table with those darn photographs. I dared to take a lunch break. I was banging pots and pans. Tom said nothing. He knew I was angry about something because of all the racket I was making. Yah, I'm mad all right. There

Impossible Choices

are so many pictures, and I'm angry with myself for having let them accumulate without putting them into photo albums. Tom came in from playing with Kara and asked, "Why the rush? Where do you think you're going?" I just thought to myself, should have done this a long time ago. Why on earth do folks procrastinate on these sorts of projects, allowing them to become avalanches? Ugh! Just keep going—and I did.

Tom has taken Kara out for the afternoon and left me to undertake the organization of years worth of snapshots. I'm taking a little writing break here; I've received many calls from our family and friends including many of the women in my support group. They've been asking questions; most of which I don't seem to be able to answer. Everyone is wondering what's really going on. I wish I knew myself. Imagine my dismay! I still can't believe this is happening.

January 11, 1999

Monday... back to work with a bang! I arrived at my desk so fatigued from lack of sleep that I couldn't concentrate. Still no word on the results from the blood work, chest scan, or abdominal scan from Friday, and it's now after four o'clock in the afternoon. I phoned the surgeon's office and asked that I have a call back with the results. This waiting is killing me. Will I ever get used to the deprivations I am forced to endure?

It wasn't until evening that she called to report that no soft tissue such as my liver or lungs, has signs of metastasis. I was relieved to say the least, but I'm not going to sleep much better tonight thinking about the bone scan scheduled for tomorrow. These are all important tests, but this scan is the one in question. After reporting my anxiety to her, the doctor has assured me that I will get a wet reading the same day so I won't have to wait for the results again.

January 12, 1999
Both Tom and Kim took today off from work to be with me. They are experts at small talk and managed to distract me a bit. Tom gave me a greeting card which never left my hands. I even asked that I lay it beneath me during the test. My Hallmark has a beautiful rainbow on the front and it reads, "I believe in miracles and dreams come true!" Tom added his own message about believing in me and that we will have a miracle.

After the scan, the three of us remained in the waiting area for the preliminary news. I was nauseous and hardly able to keep track of the conversation. Kim and Tom were at it again, their voices a bit muffled in my head. Though I sat between them, I couldn't tell you what they were saying. The nurse appeared an hour later and announced the scan was normal. I immediately broke into tears and hugged Tom and Kim. Right there in the waiting area I sobbed the happiest tears. Even the nurse Gwen got a strong hug. I asked to have the surgeon call me because I still had a lot of unanswered questions.

This evening the doctor phoned again, this time with a few brief explanations that didn't add up. My biggest uncertainty is why the scan in July showed hot spots when the scan today was clean. The doctor said the scan is so sensitive it could have picked up an injury. Hmmm... but I don't remember falling or hurting myself. The conversation was brief and she advised me to see my oncologist on Thursday as a follow-up. This appointment with the oncologist was made when we thought the cancer had spread to my bones. Hmmm... and the surgeon still wants me to keep it? Okay.

Impossible Choices

January 14, 1999

Off to the oncologist for a now "routine" follow-up to this very bad scare. She began the visit by telling me how she couldn't believe what happened. All the while, I was thinking yes, it was quite an ordeal. She continued by apologizing about the mix-up. Dumfounded I asked whatever was she speaking of? ... What? Those bone scans belong to another patient? Are you kidding? Evidently the surgeon had her own doubts about the discrepancy with the two scans and did some research! In the end, an investigation of the original report disclosed the error! The wrong results were dictated by the radiologist to my medical record number! And the wrong result was filed inside my chart at the surgeon's office! The surgeon had phoned me at home this morning but I had already left for work and had missed the call. So no, I wasn't aware of anything of the sort! My first reaction was happiness actually. Well, that explains everything. I'm going to be okay, how lucky I am! My oncologist went on with her very sympathetic apology. Her words were genuine. She was deeply sorry about what I had just been through. I left her office feeling no remorse. Here she was apologizing and she had nothing to do with it. I was just so relieved the cancer was not back.

However, I went home to that message from the surgeon on my answering machine. Her voice was almost cavalier as it recorded. I listened and heard: "Mrs. Dooling you are perfectly fine. The bone scan in July belonged to a different patient and you are just fine."

I began to ponder this past week and how horrific it had been. I tried to piece everything together. Back in July, six months prior to this mess, I saw my surgeon because I was having pain in my arm which I thought was related to the lumpectomy. Nearly one year

Barbara Dooling

out from the procedure, I continued to get this unexplained pain in that arm. A bone scan was ordered by the surgeon to rule out metastatic disease. As always, I phoned the office for the result and I was definitely told it was normal. If I was told otherwise, don't you think they would have said and done something about it?! My God, of course they would have! And so would have I.

So, there was a terrible error made at the Mass General that involved me! The bone scan result was confused with another woman's! Unfortunately, this other report was given to me and I had to undergo all kinds of tests and a week of pure hell, and I get no explanation from my surgeon, the one who ordered the test in the first place? Is this all true? After thinking things over, I began to feel that this surgeon needed to explain everything very clearly so I could process this better. I also wanted to hear if the staff in both the radiology department and the surgeon's office had been alerted to the mishap so more caution would be taken in the future. I felt that everyone should know what happened so that they could learn from the experience—changing a negative to a positive. The hope that this example might prevent another woman from suffering the same hell was a silver lining to my grievous, unnecessary ordeal. I had lost confidence in my physician, and I knew I could not continue my relationship with her unless we cleared the air. I debated changing care at this hospital, but hoped that there was a better solution. Until this point, I felt my care had been excellent, and the doctors who treated me for breast cancer were a fine team. I am also aware that mistakes can happen anywhere.

The message on my machine indicated that the surgeon was not going to call me back and I was not scheduled to see her again. She just suggested I follow-up with my medical oncologist. Tomorrow, I will arrange a meeting to speak with this surgeon. I'm

Impossible Choices

not letting this go. She hasn't even apologized!

It is most disturbing that it appeared the surgeon never saw the results of the bone scan that she ordered for me. Surely if she had, she would have questioned the possible metastasis. Again, because no one explained the error to me, it's unclear how it all happened. I also wonder whatever happened to the poor woman who actually had the abnormal result. Did she get a normal reading and go untreated? I know that I'll never find that out. I can only speculate on what happened. Certainly the misinterpretation should have been discovered six months ago. Furthermore, it was conveyed to me by an assistant that the results were normal, yet there in the chart was a report of suspicious metastatic disease. More tests were warranted at the time. If the cancer was in my bones, I would need to be treated right away to prevent further spread to the bones and to soft tissue like the liver. What a mess!

January 19, 1999

Wow, people I know are coming out with all kinds of advice on what they would do if this had happened to them. I've got quite a collection of lawyers' names. No, that isn't my answer. I need to handle the situation myself. I want to continue my relationship with my doctor because I feel she's a good surgeon.

I must make that appointment with her so we can talk face-to-face. I feel that there was negligence regarding two principal errors during my medical care. All I'm looking for is an explanation and a sincere apology, both of which I haven't received from the surgeon. She did not make the actual errors, however I was under her care at the time, she had ordered the test, and the incorrect result was provided to her office. Again, I wonder if she even saw the result. Furthermore, there's been no recognition of the terrible anxiety my family and I suffered before the results of the repeated bone scan. I'm more upset about the lack of compassion and how the problem has been handled than I am about the actual error. I realize mistakes happen and human error is unavoidable. Unfortunately, the stakes are higher in medicine. The consequences of those inaccuracies can be enormous.

February 5, 1999

Alas, today I had the meeting with my surgeon. I spoke to several staff members, nurses and secretaries, to inquire if they had been informed about the problem within the office. It bothers me tremendously that not one person that I questioned knew. Quite the contrary, everything was hushed!

When a nurse announced my name for my appointment, she automatically guided me to an examining room. I was kind but direct when I requested to see the surgeon in her office, as I was not there to be examined. I remained very calm when I spoke with my doctor. I carefully chose my words. My voice was strong and direct. We talked for forty minutes before I felt that I had finally made her understand what I expected from her as a human being, not even as my doctor. I explained that my resentment toward her was because of her coldness. I never once raised my voice, angry as I was. And I never used inappropriate language.

The surgeon told me she would understand perfectly if I chose to change health care providers. She went on to explain how much time and effort she had put into this case. I told her that I respected the strict detail she had given, but that I expected no less. Someone had to straighten out the matter.

When I asked for specifics about the error, she responded that part of the problem was that my chart had been missing so that documentation of who gave me the results was not available. Okay, now my record was missing?! We came to a standstill on the explanation. I accepted that for some reason. I asked her for some recognition of how she thought I must have felt throughout the ordeal. I asked her why she never apologized to me or expressed her own thoughts about what had happened. I gave her my opinion: that patients are people who want to be treated with compassion, especially by their doctors. To this my doctor did tell me that she regretted what had happened and no one was sorrier than her. We shook hands and I believe my doctor has learned a great deal from the experience. Yes, she is still my doctor.

I learned something as well. I realize that doctors can be wrong. They are people just like me; they are not gods! I learned not to be intimidated to ask questions... how to be patient with doctors when they don't understand the emotional impact that cancer—and all the tests that go along with it—have on people. I am grateful to those doctors who do! And I learned that patients can express their anger to their doctors and still keep their doctor/patient relationship. Like any relationship in our lives, communication is essential. I believe that if I had not expressed my feelings, and given my physician an opportunity to hear my concerns, I would only be hurting myself. And I want my doctors to respect me.

This was how my New Year began! I am so thankful that the cancer has not come back! Tom and I will try to put this behind us and continue to stay positive, but it has definitely been a set back emotionally!

March 17, 1999

I'm beginning to rest a bit easier about the cancer. Trying to make the huge decision to get pregnant again. After that scare in January, Tom is reluctant to take the plunge. I can't blame him, but my feelings haven't changed. I still want another baby. At this point, I'm totally disappointed that planning for our second baby has been put on hold. The cancer hit like a tidal wave, and stopped us from doing a lot of things, but this has been the most painful one to accept.

I owe a lot to the radiologist who diagnosed the cancer. A year ago, when I started going to the breast cancer support group, I remember learning about many women who had been misdiagnosed. They had lumps in their breasts which their doctors just "watched" by following up with repeat mammograms in six months. Many of these lumps turned out to be cancerous tumors. In some cases the cancer spread to adjacent lymph nodes under the arm.

Thank goodness I questioned the lump in my breast even though on the mammogram the small nodule did not appear to be cancerous. The radiologist was ninety-eight percent sure that it was benign. I remember him saying, "Let's be one hundred percent sure." He went on to do an ultrasound of the breast and that result, too, appeared nonmalignant. Yah, I was so relieved. But the radiologist did not stop there. By doing a noninvasive needle biopsy to be absolutely sure, he found the cancer. Hmmm, we were all astonished—me, the doctor, and Tom. Thinking back, I was so lucky this radiologist pursued things in the manner he did because my cancer was aggressive.

Well, I must move forward! I need answers about a future pregnancy. Both Tom and I have lots of questions regarding the possibility of the cancer recurring. I've remained cancer-free for nearly two years now. All the while, I continuously remind the team

Impossible Choices

of doctors that we want to have another child. During treatments, we took careful steps to ensure the preservation of my fertility. So it's time to make this decision.

April 3, 1999

Little Miss Kara Elizabeth is just that—little. Despite her petite size, she is a mighty powerful child. I have seen her lift twice her weight. When she is unable to hoist an object that is too large, my pee wee drags the object just like an animal does with its kill. Yes, Kara has incredible strength! She is just over two years old now and she has mastered the large jungle gym at the park. While holding a tight grip, she climbs with such confidence. When she does stumble up the ladder, her tiny hands do not lose their hold. Her body dangles for a moment until her feet find the rung. I watch with fright.

Other parents gasp at the sight of her swinging like a monkey from overhead bars that even preschoolers have trouble mastering. When my gymnast has finished giving me, and the other adults, a few extra heart palpitations, she runs around the far edges of the park in a complete square. In all the many days we have visited the park, I have never seen any other children do such a thing. I have to jog along behind, pretending to chase her. By the second lap around the park, I'm half jogging and half walking while I try to catch my breath. One of the dads has nicknamed her "the marathon girl." She just keeps running like a wild dog that has broken loose from its chain. I suspect if she has a mind to, she will be quite an athlete one day.

April 22, 1999

What a happy birthday! I turned thirty-eight today and received the most fabulous birthday surprise... I've begun to menstruate again! How sensational is that? I feel like a teenager! Ever since the chemo stopped my periods, I've been trying to visualize my ovaries functioning again. I tried to think of an egg traveling down the fallopian tube. Sounds crazy, but my logic was that maybe mind over matter really works! No more hot flashes! Yippee! And if we should decide to have another baby, it's at least now a possibility.

May 19, 1999

Wow, I'm finding out that there is much debate over whether women should have babies after breast cancer. This still remains a disputed medical issue. Even within the past few years, women with a history of breast cancer have been greatly advised against pregnancy. Because this kind of cancer is affected by hormones, mainly estrogen, it was believed that pregnancy hormones would cause any lingering cancer cells to flare-up.

I have attended several seminars and talks on the subject and have found few answers. Some of the finest and most respected physicians are unable to agree on any positive interpretation for medical advice. Medical experts continue trying to prove this theory one way or the other. In my search for information, I have been told it is a theory that has not been well studied. Just my luck!

June 9, 1999

We started Kara in ballet and tap lessons back in September. The recital is in ten days. Bless the teacher; she is a lovely person and has such patience with the children. Today Miss Janice opened the blinds on the big window for all the moms to view dance class. Kara is quite the ballerina. She calls herself a "balla-bina," and she is most serious. I have enjoyed watching her balance on those small feet

Impossible Choices

while she tries ever so hard to keep her hands clasped above her head. I am confident that she will not topple off the stage during her recital. She is just so adorable in that tutu. I have refrained from bringing the video camera to the classes, but today I did take some photographs. Kara is the littlest dancer in the group. Her friends are taller and much bigger than she. They are all precious.

July 10, 1999

I'm two years out from the wicked "C" word and my oncologist gave me her blessing to pursue getting pregnant! She has advised us to wait two to five years, preferably five. The longer I remain in remission, the less chance of the cancer coming back. My decision is made. I want to get pregnant providing Tom is ready, too. I will always have regrets if I let the cancer hold us back. I'd like to wait the five years, but gosh, I'm thirty-eight. I just don't want to have difficulty conceiving.

August 22, 1999

Tom and I have decided to wait another few months and take a rest from all the stress created by this decision. We won't do anything just yet. I'm two years in remission. I can wait a bit longer. Though we've complied with my oncologist's advice, the cancer still weighs heavily on our minds.

Our neighbor Nancy was pregnant with twins during the spring! I gave her all my maternity clothes to borrow. She had the babies in May—a boy and a girl. How perfect! Anyway, she returned the clothes today. Tom proceeded to store them in the attic. He asked me, "We keepin' these clothes?" And I sheepishly replied, "What do you want to do?" He climbed into the attic with the stack on his back without answering. I said, "Don't put them too far back."

Barbara Dooling

Tom poked his head from the attic and with his bright smile he said, "I won't!"

Oh, thank you, God, for letting him come around. I knew he would, I just knew he would. Well, if I'm honest with myself, I've been worried that Tom is too nervous to go forward with having another child. He is very concerned! But he does seem to be softening.

August 30, 1999

Okay, so far I've visited five different hospitals to consult with physicians and to gain as much medical knowledge as I possibly can. I want to explore the issue thoroughly. Although Tom has been more than willing to attend these appointments with me, he wants me to decide what is best for my own body in relation to this cancer. Of course he feels we should make the decision together because we are both impacted emotionally by the outcome. Yet he wants me to come to terms with it mentally first, since the risk impacts me physically.

Off I went collecting all the facts by attending appointments since April. Now it's summer, and I'm still in a dither. My long list of questions is always the same. I don't want to be ignorant about my health and jeopardize my survival. By seeking all these opinions, I'm not trying to "doctor hop" to find a physician who will pat me on the back and say, "go for it, everything will be fine." I'm wise enough to know that no one is going to give me that confirmation. I'm merely trying to educate myself on this complex and controversial issue. And I have learned something different from each specialist.

The same information kept coming from their lips; it's a theory not proven. There are studies which have been printed in medical journals showing that women who became pregnant after breast

Impossible Choices

cancer have done no worse than those who did not get pregnant. This is when there was no recurrence of the disease while they were pregnant. However those who were pregnant and did have a recurrence tended to have a worse prognosis because treatment would not be as vigorous in pregnant women. Furthermore, some women might postpone treatment or surgery until after the baby was born. Whew... what a headful. Current studies indicate that pregnancy does not cause the cancer to flare-up.

The main questions I have are:

1) If the cancer does come back while I'm pregnant, can I be given chemotherapy and will it cause birth defects?

2) If the cancer does come back, what will the course of action be and do I have a safety net to fall back on?

3) What about the chemotherapy I already had? Did this harm my eggs in any way?

4) Will I have to deliver the baby early or can I go full term?

Realistically, I know the cancer can come back. This is beginning to feel like a scary carnival ride. Once I get pregnant, there's no turning back! It will be like the roller coaster creeping up that huge hill to the top and plunging!

I was told by each physician that certain chemotherapy agents are not a concern for birth defects. And it most definitely is not a problem from the drugs I have taken in the past. There are chemo drugs that can be used, preferably after the first trimester. Considering its toxicity, I find this hard to believe. I was given the names and telephone numbers of several women who have had chemotherapy during pregnancy, and whose babies are perfectly fine. It saddens me to be asking such horrible questions, but they are absolutely necessary. The doctors have also reminded me that the chemotherapy I already had could cause problems with ovulation, thus with infertility. Hopefully I've avoided that complication by taking the Lupron injections back in 1997. Lupron suppresses ovarian function during chemo treatments. Although my periods have returned, I'm still not sure I'm actually ovulating.

During the consultations, basically each doctor gave me a firm handshake and told me how courageous I was, and wished me the best of luck. I don't feel very brave at all. I am terrified! I'm a pioneer with this journey. I just want to go on with my life. Tom and I keep agonizing over our decision. Doctors keep telling me there is no right or wrong choice here, just a very personal one. I run the risk of the cancer coming back anyway, and I must ask myself, am I going to leave two children to grow up without their mother? Then I overcome that thought by telling myself I want Kara to have a sibling. I do not want her to be alone in this world. All the relatives and friends are not going to be the same as a sibling. I believe in my heart that I must go on as if I am healthy. I cannot look back!

September 11, 1999

The summer has quickly come to an end with temperatures dropping and the first cool days setting in. Today we picked plump juicy apples from the brimming orchards. The trees stood firm and secure, but their branches drooped with heavy ripe fruit. I plucked a single red apple and pretended to be Eve in the garden of Eden. I held my temptation out to Tom, and with seducing eyes, I ordered him to take a bite. If it were not for Kara and the other pickers, I am certain he would have taken more than that bite right there on the grass. We settled for a sensuous kiss. Kara delighted in running in and out of the maze, and stumbled many times on the fallen apples that littered the ground. We laughed at her clumsiness.

Impossible Choices

Kara keeps asking for a brother or sister. I suppose lots of kids do at her age. She'll be three in November. I'm pushing thirty-nine. What to do, what to do. What would you do? I have been praying fiercely for God to send me an answer.

October 3, 1999

I watch Kara play with her baby dolls as she tucks them snugly under a blanket. She kisses her two babies and tells them to dream sweet dreams. Next she pats their heads and flips them over to rub their backs. I hear her whisper, "I love you, OHHHH much." My eyes fill with tears. She amazes me. I am careful not to disturb her and the babies. I continue listening. Hmm… today is Alicia's birthday. Happy Birthday, Alicia Marie.

October 6, 1999

A visit to Nana and Grandpa's house this afternoon. Mommy has been eager to show Kara-Girl a surprise. Today, we shall take Mommy's old bedroom set for my sweet little Kara. I ask her, "Do you like the set?" And she answers, "Mommy, dis you room?" Yes, Darling, it was Mommy's set, and now it's yours.

I am glad to see her get the bedroom, but I shall be ever so sad to see my baby girl leave the crib. I want to mother and nurture her forever. I guess mommies are like that, Kara. I suppose some things never change.

October 12, 1999

How funny Kara-Girl was today! You have a little head cold and Mommy tried to help you blow your nose. Kara got angry and told Mommy, "I want my boogies. Don't you take them." Well, Kara, I nearly fell over laughing. You would not blow your nose for me.

Barbara Dooling

Fine, Miss Kara, you keep your boogers! Kara sneezes and says, "You bless me, Mommy?" Yes, God bless you, Kara. Happy Birthday, Geno.

October 15, 1999

Pizza-face Kara usually wears more than she eats. Friday night pizza and Daddy stopped at the library for a movie. It's a cold fall evening, and the Dooling bears are snug inside watching "Bambi." My bear cub sits on Mommy's lap through the whole show. I reach around and squeeze her then hold her tiny hands in mine. Seems my girly-girl is getting so big. Daddy sends me over a wink!

October 17, 1999

Sunday. Kara came into the kitchen to tell Mommy, "I go sit in my time out chair." First time she ever announced that! I proceeded into the living room in haste to investigate. The couch had been newly decorated with bright colors. The hardwood floor and her toy chest lavishly colored as well. Seems Kara-Girl found the crayons that have been put away for this very reason. I guess coloring on paper is not as much fun. Mommy shouted and Kara got frightened. She called out from her chair, "You angry, Mommy?" I answer, "Yes, Kara, but we can clean this up. I still love you, and I'm sorry for raising my voice and frightening you."

Poor little Kara got scolded again for the graffiti. Daddy saw the mess and gave her a sponge to scrub the floor. She refused to put the scrubbing pad in her hand, claiming, "But Dad, I'm only little and I can't do it." Daddy and I chuckled. He told her to get cleaning and I had to leave the room for fear I would burst into laughter.

She looked like the sorriest little girl.

Impossible Choices

October 19, 1999

This evening Kara must be thinking about her great artwork. Daddy finally managed to remove the stains from the couch. Kara was curiously running her hands over the exact spot where the marks had been. She pulled out a piece of white paper from the stash and quietly asked, "I have the crayons, Mommy? I write on paper. I no write on the couch." Mom had to think about this one… I decided that she'd already had several chances. I said no to my artist. Kara yelled out, "I not writing on the floor, Mommy. I not. I promise I not." That's correct, Sweet Pea, you won't have the chance.

October 21, 1999

Mommy and Daddy were being silly tonight and woke Kara up by accident. Daddy threw his extra heavy weight pillow at me and knocked me down. That pillow can scarcely be called a headrest. I get a nosebleed if I turn over and bump it during my sleep. We were laughing so hard that Kara woke up in a delirious state. Sorry, Girly-Girl. Mommy put you back to bed. As I tucked Kara in, I found Daddy's picture and his shirt on her pillow. Kara always loves to cuddle up with Daddy's shirt instead of her stuffed bear. Kara-Girl sure loves her Daddy! Me, too!

October 22, 1999

Another attempt to find your crayons. Wherever did Mommy hide them? You are a persistent little girl!

October 24, 1999

Tom and I celebrated our fifth wedding anniversary this month. We traveled to the Balsams Resort in Dixville Notch, New

Barbara Dooling

Hampshire, five hours from Boston. It was truly lovely and Karaless. Tee hee hee, tee hee. We stayed two nights at this grand place while Kara enjoyed the cottage in Maine with Grammy and Grampy Dooling. My in-laws are wonderful to have given us this time together. When we got back to Melrose, Tom and I renewed our wedding vows! That's right, why wait till your twenty-fifth or fiftieth for this celebration?

When I think back to October 1994, I remember our wedding day was so joyous. Now I can think back on renewing our vows. If I had my way, I'd get married every year! Our parish priest thought it was very romantic to renew our vows. We enjoyed the day with a simple ceremony at St. Mary's church. Uncle Howie officiated the service. I surprised Tom and Kara with a white horse drawn carriage just like the one we had on our first wedding day. We had a perfectly wonderful two hour ride through Melrose and around two ponds in the area. The foliage was bursting with vibrant colors on this warm Indian summer day. I wore my going away suit. Yes, it still fits! Before we rode through the wooded part of Melrose along the ponds, we trotted right down Main Street. Kara was squealing with laughter and waving to everyone! My, what a pleasant day.

October 28, 1999

We have had a very mild fall thus far. The days have been just lovely. Foliage has peaked here in Melrose and the colors are brilliant despite the lack of rain this past summer. The sky is clear and blue with white fluffy clouds drifting off to the South. They are well-defined cumulus that form elephants, rabbits, and turtles in the sky. It is refreshing to wallow in such a wonderful day. I have a lighthearted feeling. The passing of summer is never a loss for me because autumn is my favorite time of year. The season is alive even

Impossible Choices

though it brings the harvest and hibernation. This change in seasons is thought to be the end of many things. When the leaves turn russet, they fall from the trees leaving them bare and lifeless. However, autumn commands refreshing cool days after the steaming heat of summer. For me, it is a splendid time of year.

November 5, 1999

Daddy and Kara-Girl make a messy but delicious pizza. I think there is more sauce on you and dad than on the pizza. While we wait for our meal prepared by the great chefs of Melrose, I jot this quick entry while you and Daddy play tickles on the floor. Dad is chasing you around the furniture. You look like two squirrels circling a tree trunk. You are laughing so hard that your face is red and sweaty. You've started a new game. You are galloping on your dad. He makes a fine horsy. Using his ears for reins, you pull back and say, "Giddy up!" Poor Daddy shouts in pain. Daddy is no longer amused with you in the saddle; he gives one good buck. Off you go!

November 12, 1999

I sing my Kara to sweet slumber trying my best to stay in tune with the song you chose. Lucky for me you are too young or too sleepy to notice I do not harmonize well. I am more than a bit off-key. The noisy autumn wind is whirling about outside, rattling the windows. The house is chilly and I tuck your tiny body snug inside your Pooh bear quilt. You are so content. I love you, Kara Elizabeth! I love you! Happy Birthday, Russ.

November 18, 1999

Kara turned threeeeeeeeeeeeee today! We had a great party for her with the three bears and Goldilocks, too. We cooked homemade

Barbara Dooling

beef stew and chicken soup, inviting folks over for porridge. My Kara-Girl is full of ginger and spice, vinegar and vigor. She never walks. She always runs. My girly-girl is tenacious and determined, keen and intelligent. She is a character in every way, dramatic and comical. Kara-Cub is very tiny yet she is are very, very strong! Yup, she is really something else! Happy Birthday, Kara Elizabeth and Uncle Kenny.

November 21, 1999

We attend the christening of Mommy's great-nephew, baby Kevin. Kara is excited to see so many babies. You love the beautiful white gowns they wear. Kara asks, "Where our baby, Mom?" I point to our guest of honor, but you insist he is not our baby. You are more specific and explain, "Mommy's, and Daddy's baby." Maybe someday, Bear Cub. Maybe soon we'll have a baby.

November 22, 1999

Kara is helping in the kitchen again! Mommy is making Daddy's favorite pumpkin bread for Thanksgiving. You like to crack the eggs. Very few shells in the batter this time, I'm impressed. Daddy says no one will know if they are shells or nuts. He is a nut! Happy Birthday, Tyla Marie.

November 23, 1999

Today we visit Grandpa for his birthday. Kara insists that the cake is for her. You're smart, Kara, because your birthday was only less than a week ago. Nana pampers you with her famous Chickerina Soup! You devour the tiny meatballs and Nana loves to watch you eat! Happy Birthday, Dad.

Impossible Choices

November 28, 1999

We decorate the house for Christmas! Kara is amazed at all the "stuff" we have. Daddy has rock music blasting on the stereo. Mommy persuades him to put on some Christmas tunes. I tell Dad the Christmas songs put me in the mood. Daddy says, "I'm always in the mood." Silly Daddy—he is.

December 4, 1999

Off to pick out a Christmas tree today. Kara has more fun running in and out among the trees which are lined like a holly maze. You keep asking, "Daddy, you like dis one?" Daddy shouts, "That's too big!" And Mommy pipes up, "It's perfect, I love it!" We get the big one just like every year. Poor daddy struggles to get it inside the house. He complains, "It's too big!" Mommy chuckles to herself—careful not to let him see her smiling. It's perfect!

December 7, 1999

We begin to decorate the very large Christmas tree. The lights are so beautiful. Kara is delighted with the festivities. We play Christmas music and Daddy puts in the movie video, *It's a Wonderful Life.* So much going on all at once, but that's Christmas! Happy Birthday, Christopher Edward.

December 9, 1999

Oh how Kara enjoys the decorations about the house and on the tree! Her favorite are the gold jingle bells. She collected as many of these chimes that would fit inside her tea set. Eventually they make it back on the tree. Kara puts them all on the same branch. It is weighed down by so many ornaments. That is Kara's branch, and she pings the bells each time she walks by.

Barbara Dooling

We have a lovely nativity set on the buffet. Mommy has explained the word "Fragile" to Kara. We learn about baby Jesus who you have mistakenly named baby Moses. That's a different book, Kara. Anyway, baby whoever was missing. I found him wrapped in a kitchen towel with a tiny white baby bottle beside him. We carefully set baby Jesus back in the manger. When I was a little girl, Kara, Mommy used to play with Nana's baby Jesus, too.

December 10, 1999
Mommy is spellbound by the beauty of our Christmas tree. The collection of ornaments is just spectacular. We talk about Santa Claus and the traditional Christmas fun. Kara keeps saying that Santa will bring her everything. Daddy and I explain this is not so. You tell Mommy, "Call Santa on the phone for me. I want you to call Santa." I guess you figured out how to go right to the source!

December 11, 1999
Today we visit grandpa in the hospital. Kara graciously offers her teddy bear to make him feel better. Grandpa tucks him into bed with him. When we leave, you ask, "Grandpa, you done wit my bear? I need to take him home wit me. He a missin' me." We all laughed. You were very kind and generous to share your bear with Grandpa.

December 14, 1999
Answering the telephone is such fun these days. We have been teaching Kara to ask, "Who is it, please?" She has become quite the secretary stating, "Dis is Kara Duuuulin and who you?" Tonight Kara answers one phone, and I pick up the other in the kitchen. I realize it is a sales call and gently hang the phone up allowing her to chat. Eventually, the person gives up hope of speaking with an adult and

Impossible Choices

hangs up. Mommy has a good laugh.

December 17, 1999

Back to Santa's list. She has been asking for a real baby. Mommy would love for Kara to have a brother or sister. Oh my sweet, Bear Cub, I would love that.

December 20, 1999

We are preparing for the big day. Lots of talk about Santa's arrival and the birth of baby Jesus. More play with the nativity. Kara keeps taking the shepherd's staff and calling it "hook." I agreed with you that it did look like a hook. You corrected me and said, "Just like Captain Hook in Peter Pan." Wow, what an observation! You're my smart girly-girl!

December 21, 1999

Your annual pediatric exam—three year check up. The doctor plays a little game with you while she looks inside your ears. She is meowing like a cat and asking if you have a kitten inside your ear. Kara corrected the doctor in a most confident voice and said, "There no kitty in my ear. I have a drum." The doctor was astonished.

December 22, 1999

Kara has been searching the skies for Santa at night. You ask, "Where is he, mommy? When is he coming?" I understand it's hard to wait, My Darling. You look so adorable as you press your nose to the cold window pane and gaze out into the darkness. I love you, my precious lamb.

Barbara Dooling

December 24, 1999

A surprise visit from Santa this evening! He came rushing through the back door with a sack full of toys. What a surprise for Kara! He actually came to our house to make sure this is where Kara lived. She was not frightened in the least. She leaped off the couch like a cat and ran to Santa shouting, "Oh, Santa, I love you!" With the greatest of hugs, her tiny arms tried to wrap around Santa's fat waist. Mommy got teary-eyed. Our jolly guest hoisted Kara onto his lap and asked the famous question.

You gladly sat on his lap and recited your wish-list. You told Santa you wanted a baby. Santa asked if you wanted a baby dolly. To this you corrected Santa and said, "Not a dolly, I want a real baby. I want a brother or sister." Santa started to leave, saying he'd be back later with the heavy stuff. And Kara shouted, "I live right here, Santa. Right here in this house with my mommy and daddy." You didn't forget that he said that he was trying to find you.

We set out cookies and milk for him, a whole lot of carrots for his reindeer, and kissed baby Jesus good night. Mommy told Kara that tomorrow was baby Jesus' birthday. Lucky the little fellow is still in one piece since Kara keeps stealing him from the hay. How she marvels at that tiny porcelain baby.

We marched upstairs and peeked out the window to have a look for Santa in the sky, but we did not see him. Off to bed everybody... and all Christmas wishes will come true.

December 25, 1999

Merry Christmas, Kara, my darling angel. Merry, Merry Christmas Daddy Tom. Happy birthday, baby Jesus. What a delightful morning. Our precious Kara is full of excitement and grinning with joy. How amazed she was upon entering the living room to see such

Impossible Choices

an array of colorful packages under the tree. Some of the items are unwrapped, and she runs to them immediately! Kara asks Mommy how Santa could carry all these toys in one small sleigh. Gosh, her smart mind is always going. Santa brought wooden furniture for Kara's dolls. There's a cradle with a pastel quilt, a highchair with a teddy bear propped inside the seat, an armoire with tiny outfits hanging inside, and a small rocking chair with a kitty sitting on it. These were openly displayed under the tree. What a lucky girl you are! As you tear open the remaining packages, Mommy and Daddy snuggle together on the couch.

The best gift of all was yet to come. Mommy took a home pregnancy test, and we got a real baby! Mommy is going to have a baby! Daddy is going to have another cowgirl or cowboy to ride his back! Kara, you're going to have a brother or sister! Yep, Mommy and Kara's wish was the same and we got a real baby! We're pregnant! We're pregnant! I bought the home kit yesterday and anxiously waited until Christmas morning to do the test! Isn't it just grand? I'm going to have another baby! I love you, sweetness Kara, I love you, Tom!

We shared our wonderful news with the family later today when everyone was gathered at the table for dinner. Daddy reveals the surprise by announcing to everyone that next year there will be one more person at the table to bless.

December 30, 1999

Each night when she arrives home with her daddy, I hear such screaming coming from the driveway and all the way to the front door. Kara shouts, "Mooommmy, Moooommmmy, I home. Where are you, Moooommmy?" Yes, Kara, Mommy is home and I can hear you from all parts of the house, even the cellar. I am certain the neighbors can hear your calls, too. I drop everything and come running to greet you. I love how you keep yelling until you reach my arms. It is without a doubt my favorite part of the day!! It really is a wonderful life. I love you, Kara.

December 31, 1999

New Year's Eve! A new millennium on its way. Kara, you were snug in your bed while Mommy and Daddy watched the celebration around the world on TV. We held hands while we kissed and thanked each other and God for our millennium baby! And we thanked God for our little Kara-Girl.

January 7, 2000 Millennium News

Today I have a whole day to myself so I can sit down and write guilt-free in my journal. There is plenty to do in this house—cleaning and such. Instead, I'm going to indulge in my thoughts and roam the pages of a lifetime here in this book filled with dates and events.

Outside the wind is howling on this frigid day; but I am warm and cozy inside my messy house. Wind gusts are shifting the small loose items in the back yard from one side to the next. Trash cans are rolling around and the gas grill cover has been shredded in half. It too, is whirling about. Woah Nelly! There goes the bird house right into our neighbor's yard. I keep getting distracted by all the noises. This old house is creaking and seems to be almost moving with the gale forces. Hope all the homeless people have sought shelter somewhere. I feel so happy and safe to be here in my little house on such a blustery day.

I just can't believe I'm going to have another baby! Since the first day I learned I had breast cancer, I prayed to God that Tom and

Impossible Choices

I and Kara would not be deprived of a precious baby to complete our family. Actually, I remember before I even knew I had cancer, when Kara was just six months old, Tom and I started talking about getting pregnant again. Yep, we were planning to have children close together because I was thirty-five when I had Kara, and we feared the infertility scene. I was so fortunate to become pregnant on the first try with Kara. And then, because of the chemotherapy I had in 1997, we weren't sure if the chemotherapy stopped me from ovulating.

That day in the radiologist's office when I was first diagnosed with breast cancer, I just cried and cried because I wanted another baby. He was very encouraging about future pregnancies, though he suggested that I take things one step at a time. I believe that it was this little tiny piece of hope from my doctor, and my lifelong dream of the perfect family, and my intense bond to my husband and girly-girl Kara, that pulled me through the cancer so miraculously. See how dreams can save your life?

For the Dooling family, it will be an extra special new year... we are celebrating our good news, our good fortune, and our good health.

January 8, 2000

Daddy is mercilessly tickling Kara on the living room floor. He offers her a short break and allows her to go free. As she carefully walks away, she throws a glance over her shoulder in a most untrusting way. Before she can reach the safety of the couch, Daddy's fast, strong arms capture Kara and pull her back down to the floor. What a shriek she lets out as he repeats this again and again. He is relentless, but it is evident how much she loves this game.

Barbara Dooling

January 11, 2000

You have redesigned the toy box again. This time you have chosen a lovely bright orange and red to scribble across the entire lid. Daddy said no more crayons, pens, pencils, and markers for the rest of your life!

January 12, 2000

Mommy's first prenatal exam since the news of her pregnancy. I come home full of information for Daddy. Kara listens to our conversation and claims that Daddy has a baby in his belly, too. We carefully explain that girls have babies, not boys. You are quite pleased about this and ask, "I have a baby in my tummy, Mommy?" No, my bear cub, just mommy has the baby.

January 20, 2000

Daddy and Kara enjoy a "Daddy-Daughter Day" walking in the woods. He made quite an adventure for you. He pretended you were exploring an Indian village with teepees, deer, rocks, and more! I hear all about your travels at dinner. I'm sorry that Mommy had to work today and couldn't join you, but it is good for you to have this time alone with your daddy. What a lucky girl you are to have such a wonderful daddy. He loves you very much and enjoys his time with you. I am a lucky girl, too, because I have both of you.

January 26, 2000

Mommy's belly is beginning to swell. We have told Kara very little about the pregnancy because the baby won't be here for a long time. She has been full of questions about my round tummy. At night, she rubs my belly and talks to our baby. Kara is excited to be

Impossible Choices

a big sister and it shows during her play with her dollies. She will positively be such a wonderful helper. I can't wait.

January 28, 2000

It is difficult to explain how our baby grows inside Mommy's belly, but Kara is catching on. She has been careful not to kick me during our rough play. This evening she included our baby in her prayers. I was astonished that she actually thought to mention baby.

January 29, 2000

Daddy is growing concerned about Mommy's growing tummy. He is worried we might be having twins because I am much bigger with this pregnancy. The doctor explains this is all quite normal during a second pregnancy. Mommy would love to have twins! Although this would surely take much more attention away from our Kara. Wish I met your daddy when I was younger. I would love to have had more children. I am thankful for you, Kara. And I am grateful that you will have a brother or sister. I am happy for you, bear cub.

January 31, 2000

My precious Kara, this year holds much promise for us! Mommy cries happy tears over the pregnancy. I am overjoyed and waiting anxiously to feel movement from your brother or sister. I remember the first time I felt you move. It was a fluttering sensation. How amazing and exciting to have life inside me! There is no finer feeling! It is miraculous! You, my tiny girl, were a very active baby. You would make me laugh and even cry whenever I felt you move about. I had the most wonderful pregnancy. I never cared that my belly was getting bigger and bigger as you grew inside me. I felt

Barbara Dooling

beautiful, radiant, and even sexy.

February 9, 2000

We hear our baby's heartbeat today! It is a wonder! I feel great and so full of energy. I am thankful for my many blessings.

February 14, 2000

Our usual Valentine's Day celebration, we try to get Kara off to bed early. Sorry, my sweet girl, you won't be dining with us tonight. We have cooked a fine meal and will dine with the fancy china. Mommy puts on her pretty red negligee that she got as a wedding gift. It is silky and glittery with appliqué and pearls. Mom's belly is big, and the gown barely fits. Daddy says I look more beautiful in it than ever before. He rubs my belly and talks to baby.

February 19, 2000

Dad and Kara-Girl go sledding at the golf course. Mommy has a sore leg and must stay home. I am disappointed to miss out on the excitement. You both come home soaking wet. I give you a hot bath and put you down for a nap. My girl is full of contentment and smiles sleepily at me. You drift off to never land as you rest your head on my belly which serves well as a pillow. I scarcely move because I am loving this moment. You are clinging to me and our baby. I gently stroke your flushed cheek. I would love to bend over and kiss that tiny nose. Though I am tempted, I do not move because I do not want to wake you. How cheerful I am this day. I love you, snuggle bear.

February 20, 2000

Daddy and I take Kara to a nearby farm—a place we have

Impossible Choices

enjoyed many times in the past. We pat the horses and goats. Though the trees appear lifeless with their bare limbs, the animals are outside on this winter day because the sun is strong and warm. Noisy children are sledding on a nearby hill. We walk around the grounds, but mommy is hobbling. That leg is no better. Kara is helpful and pushes me from behind. She runs a little bit ahead and shouts, "Mommy, I wait for you to catch up!"

February 26, 2000

Today my Kara-Girl asked mommy how the baby gets out of my belly. Wow, how do you think of these things? Kara gets her brief, for-three-year-olds version of the birds and bees. *Winnie The Pooh* and the honey tree are not included.

February 27, 2000

We dig out your baby pictures, a favorite pastime for Kara and Mommy. I am thinking back to those joyous days when I held you in my arms. You were such a tiny baby. Today you are a little girl. How quickly you have grown. I am yearning for the day our baby is born when I shall hold another babe, and you shall hold your sister or brother. I'm feeling great and enjoying every moment of my second pregnancy. Same as with you, little Kara, I feel wonderful. How fortunate to fulfill this lifelong dream. How many sacrifices have I made to make this dream come true? I'm elated. You're going to be a terrific older sister. How loving and caring you are with your dolls and stuffed animals. Perhaps all children are, but I often hear you say the sweetest things to the little people in your little world. You are always lining them up, making sure they have soft blankets and plenty of pretend food to eat. It pleases me when you tell our neighbors and friends that you are going to be a big sister. I love

Barbara Dooling

you, Bunnykins.

February 29, 2000

Kara loves animals and I'm so glad because Mommy does, too! She is learning to be gentle with all critters, domestic and wild. Mommy teaches her to be cautious, too. I believe furry creatures can teach children about love, responsibility, and even death. I have always felt this way.

March 1, 2000

I'm really showing now! My belly is popping right out. In fact, I look as though I were five months pregnant instead of four. Kara is full of questions about my protruding mound. Both she and Daddy rub my belly all the time. At night, Kara includes her baby brother/sister in her prayers. She recites, "God bless Mommy, God bless Daddy, my Nana and my Grandpa, my Grammy and my Grampy, all my cousins and God bless… Jenna Rose. She always forgets the boy's name. I tell her, Kyle Thomas if we have a boy. For some reason, she cannot remember the name Kyle. She has also renamed one of her dollies Jenna Rose. I'm beginning to wonder if Kara knows something that we don't because we're not going to find out the sex of the baby. There are so few surprises in life, we've decided to wait, wait, wait until the end, end, end. Also, during Kara's bedtime prayers, she actually remembers to ask God to make Mommy's leg all better. I'm beginning to have some hip and leg pain and I've started to limp a little bit. It's become increasingly difficult to sit and play on the floor with Kara, so naturally, she wants Mommy to get better real fast. I'm pushing thirty-nine and I guess my body is questioning this pregnancy.

Impossible Choices

March 3, 2000

It is an unseasonably warm weekend away in Maine. We head right for the beach where you and Daddy chase waves. I sit and watch my beautiful family. I am so delighted watching you, even as you get soaking wet. Let's not forget it is still March and not July. We hurry home to get into dry clothes. Daddy lights the blaze in the wood stove. I worry about you burning yourself, but Daddy is more trusting than I. Mommy reviews the wood stove rules. The stove has a glass front, and we watch the colorful flames as they warm us. I love you, precious lamb.

March 4, 2000

This evening Kara is pooped, and she is in bed by seven. She played hard today. Daddy and I sit by the fire. It is so hot we take our clothes off! Daddy is hugging Mommy's big belly. Oops, unexpected company; it's Daddy's cousin Jay and his wife Tracy. We must scramble for our clothes! The passion had to wait until our guests went home, but the laughs and pleasant conversation we shared with them were worth it.

March 5, 2000

Home today but not before visiting our deer friends. That's deer friends, not dear friends. Tee hee hee. Kara loves to stand and watch these graceful animals.

March 8, 2000

How very independent Kara is getting. Mommy is sad because I will always think of you as my baby girl. It is difficult to allow you space, but I give it to you reluctantly. I know that a mother must watch her child stumble and fall sometimes. But you are my baby girl and I want to protect you. You want to do everything yourself. Thank goodness, you still love to be cuddled and kissed. During this surge of independent behavior, you are quite verbal and tenacious. It has been the battle of the wills lately. Kara shows her angry face. It is a great angry face, but I'd much rather see that happy smile! I love you, Bunny.

March, 9, 2000

I've sought medical advice about this leg pain from my orthopedic doctor. Wow, it's really hurting and seems to be getting worse. My ortho wants me to immediately schedule an MRI given my history with the breast cancer. But I'm full of questions about the effects of an MRI on the baby. She has assured me that an MRI is not only safe during pregnancy, but it's actually used at times to diagnose problems with the fetus.

March 10, 2000

I did make that appointment, and despite the doctor's reassurance, I canceled! I called the orthopedic and asked if we could give it a few more weeks to see if I improve. Against her wishes, she has rescheduled the MRI in just two weeks. The pain in my leg is not miraculously getting better, and I've had to physically crawl up and down the stairs on all fours. I think I'm going to have to talk myself straight into that hospital for the test. Still, I keep hoping I have the famous sciatica, which is quite common in pregnancy. After all, I seem to be so much bigger during this pregnancy. I think the baby must be sitting on a nerve. Yah, that's got to be it.

March 22, 2000

It's done. I had the MRI. As I completed my paperwork before-

Impossible Choices

hand, I had to sign a special pregnancy waiver regarding unknown risks to the fetus. I began to cry and thought I was not going to go through with the test. I asked to speak with the radiologist. Of course they sent the technician out to answer my questions. The tech was knowledgeable, but I asked again that I please speak with the radiologist. The radiologist was nice enough to come out from behind wherever they hide, and his insights settled me down enough to have the MRI. I imagined this very loud diagnostic test would somehow hurt the baby's hearing and God knows what else.

They took what is called a "limited study" so the test would not be as long. As usual, my eyes were tearing the whole time. If it hadn't been for the earplugs they gave me, I am certain my ears would have been little pools of water. I worried terribly for my unborn baby. Though he or she was insulated, I couldn't help but wonder if the baby was jumping and frightened by the extremely loud knocking. Don't forget the baby did not have the same earplugs I did.

March 24, 2000

I am crying again. Howling in fact. How do I even begin to explain about the breast cancer coming back, spreading to my bones and lung. It is for real. There is no mistake this time. The cancer is back… with a vengeance! Oh dear God, the cancer has metastasized! NO! YES it has! NO, NO, NO a thousand times, NO! Yes, it has! Tom and I have been flying high with the good news of my pregnancy. The cancer just can't come crashing into our lives like this. It just can't. NO, NO, NO!

I can't believe I'm writing this in my treasured journal again. Last night my orthopedic doctor called our house at seven o'clock and spoke to Julie who was baby-sitting. She left a message that she

Barbara Dooling

would call back again at nine. I already had an uneasy feeling. I've known this doctor for many years and I have actually worked with her professionally. I have been to her home for a yearly summer fund raiser. I knew she was well aware of my anxiety regarding the results. All was not fine, so she wanted to speak directly to me. She was so punctual calling right at nine. She asked if my husband was home, only confirming my worst fears. Tom was working but I convinced her to tell me the results of that MRI. I was standing near the couch and had not yet sat down. She proceeded to bear the news, trying to be a friend as well as my doctor. I believe she was crying. I had always thought she had a soft spot in her heart for me. It was apparent she was having great difficulty relaying the news.

Her words brought me to my knees. I was so weak that I fell right to the floor, never making it to the couch. I was shaking. She said, "There's tumor. We believe the cancer has metastasized and you're going to need a biopsy right away. If this is correct, you may need to have radiation which means, Barbara, that you will have to terminate the pregnancy." I immediately told her I would never do such a thing. I continued by explaining how we had researched this very well before even getting pregnant. I knew we had options and I wasn't going to "terminate" this pregnancy. I thought to myself, this woman has never had any children. How can she tell me to terminate my pregnancy? She has no idea. She has absolutely no idea what it feels like to have life inside of you. She was trying to save my life, but I didn't want to hear what she was telling me.

I pulled myself onto the couch and hung up the phone. Julie was sitting on the love seat crying softly. We never spoke; I just picked up the phone and telephoned Tom. He said over and over again, "No, no, I just don't believe it." He headed home right away. While I waited to be comforted in his arms, I had my obstetrician

Impossible Choices

paged. It was about ten o'clock in the evening. The doctor returned the page right away, before Tom had even gotten home. I sobbed and sobbed trying to give him as much information as I could. This OB/GYN had been my doctor since I was eighteen years old, and he had delivered Kara. He knew me very well and he knew how much this baby was wanted. He had been a part of the whole decision process about getting pregnant again. He supported my every move. Now he too talked about "terminating" the pregnancy. He explained that I had to think about Tom, Kara and myself, the family I already had. I didn't want to hear that because my family now included this baby. I kept thinking that this was the OB's baby, too, because he was taking care of it. What was he saying? Did he know what he was saying to me? I just couldn't process any of this.

Tom arrived and it was take-three… the third time I was being told I had cancer. The first time being in 1997, the second was the error in 1999, and now this. We should have been well-versed, but we weren't. Nothing can prepare you for this sort of news. When it rains, it pours. In my case, it was beginning to feel like a flood. I hadn't just rocked the boat, I had tipped it over.

While I was crying in Tom's arms, Kara woke up. She heard my yelps of pain and it frightened her. She yelled downstairs to me, "Mommy, why you crying? Don't be sad, Mommy. I am here." I fled to her as fast as I could creep up those stairs.

March 24, 2000

My orthopedic doctor has already notified my oncologist of the MRI results. Tom and I, Mary, and Kenny met with my oncologist to discuss my options. She was very frank about the pregnancy, stating she does not advise us to keep the baby if the cancer turns up in other places. Why was everyone talking this way? I had researched this before getting pregnant and no one had ever mentioned the word "termination" to me.

The MRI has revealed two lesions. I am to have a bone biopsy of these areas to confirm cancer. My oncologist informed us that the procedure will take place under the guidance of a CT scan. The lesions or tumors are located deep within my pelvic region in the iliac wing. A needle will have to be guided by the CT scan to pinpoint exact location, and then guided back out. I immediately asked about the radiation to the baby. My oncologist did her best to explain that I had to have this biopsy, and the dose of radiation to the baby will be minimal. When I asked her if the test could be done under MRI guidance, she did not think so.

This afternoon, I called the radiology department at the Mass General to find out the doctor's name who is to perform my procedure. I had her paged because I wanted to ask about the risks to the pregnancy. She explained the dose of radiation to the baby would be "about 2 rads"—whatever that means. I called my Obstetrician for his input. He explained, "You need the biopsy. It's minimal radiation to the fetus." I can't help thinking the doctors are quite certain already that the dark areas on the MRI are definitely cancer. The confirmation of the biopsy will only lead to more tests to see if the cancer has spread to my lungs or liver, which means more radiation exposure to the baby. So how many rads will it total? Now what are we talking about?

Next I paged a high risk OB/GYN at the Mass General. I had already seen this doctor for a consultation prior to getting pregnant. He's had other patients with cancer who have received chemotherapy during pregnancy. I realize now that I need this doctor to follow my pregnancy. He told me the amount of rads exposed to the fetus should be kept to a minimum of five to ten, preferably

Impossible Choices

closer to five. He also gave me hope. He agreed to meet with my oncologist, and with Tom and I to discuss saving the baby. At last someone is positive about the pregnancy!

I also called the radiologist who had originally diagnosed me back in 1997. He was the doctor who had read my first mammogram which showed the lump. Through his persistence, he found the cancer early, thus I thought highly of his opinion. He agreed to see me on Monday to review the findings on the recent MRI films. I trust his judgment completely.

March 27, 2000

Monday during the consult, the radiologist agreed with everyone else about the lesions. They did look cancerous. It was difficult to review the MRI films because we could see the baby's head quite clearly. At first Tom was so frightened to continue the pregnancy. But these films made ending the pregnancy impossible. We could actually see our baby. Tom could no longer be sheltered and retreat from this invisible but living being. The pictures altered Tom's opinion and confused his thinking.

The radiologist offered his knowledge about a new MRI machine. This particular MRI, he said, was not like the usual diagnostic MRI. He believed it could be used to do the biopsy instead of a CT scan. The special MRI was open in the center where a surgeon would normally stand to perform surgical procedures. This of course would mean no radiation to the baby. Now I was ready to jump back into an MRI machine that had frightened me so much before.

He could not remember which Boston hospital had this particular machine. When I got home, I pulled out the yellow pages and called as many MRI facilities as I could. The receptionists and I hadn't a clue what type of machine I was actually even looking for. Some would say, "Oh, yes, our MRI machines are open, making them less claustrophobic than the others." I would explain I was looking for one that was open in the center, for use during surgery. I was told over and over that MRI machines are used for diagnosing and not for surgery.

I called the hospitals in Boston, including the Mass General where I am scheduled to have the biopsy done by CT scan tomorrow. Nope, not there! Finally, at the Brigham and Woman's Hospital, someone actually knew what I was asking for. JOY of JOYS! I needed to have my doctor set everything up. Of course, to complicate matters, my oncologist is on vacation. She's unavailable for two more days. I decided if this machine was at the Brigham, they must have one at the Mass General. Again I paged the radiologist at The General who is scheduled to operate on me. I haven't heard back from her, however I figure I'll just ask tomorrow.

March 29, 2000

"Tomorrow" came as it always does and I again found myself signing my life away because of the pregnancy. I was prepped in a Johnny-gown and made ready for the bone biopsy. The nurses were all a buzz and told me they were ready for me—ready and waiting for the pregnant woman. I was crazed with anxiety.

Where's the radiologist? May I speak with her? A radiologist spoke with me, but not the one who would do the biopsy. I asked about this MRI technique to guide the needle and if there was that special machine at the Mass General. The doctor did not know of it. When I told him about the one at the Brigham, he assured me that no one was forcing me to have the procedure done with CT scan,

Impossible Choices

and I could leave on my own will. I explained that I was perfectly willing to go through with what I knew had to be done, but would prefer the MRI guidance if it were possible. I asked this doctor to call the Brigham because if they couldn't do it by MRI there, I would follow through with the CT scan procedure. I was, after all, prepped and ready to go. I did not exactly want to find out the Brigham couldn't help me and have to reschedule at the Mass General.

The radiologist did call Brigham and Woman's Hospital and came back with a name of the surgeon who might do the biopsy with MRI guidance. There would be no radiation to the baby. However, this doctor is on a conference for two more days.

I had been crying that whole morning. I looked at Tom; his face and ears were beet red. Whenever his ears get red, I know he is near meltdown. His whole face, neck, and ears were ruby red. He had been quietly standing at my side during the past two hours through this back and forth negotiating. He felt the biopsy should be done. Tom thought it might be a whole week of anxiety before we got in at the Brigham. I looked him straight in the eyes and I cried some more tears.

I said, "I can't go through with this, not when there's a chance to do it a safer way." I got dressed and Tom wheeled me out of the Mass General. That's right, wheeled me. My leg is now useless; I've been using a wheelchair to move around in the hospitals. Tom was silent the whole way down to the lobby and out to the parking garage. I thought perhaps he might wheel me straight out to Storrow Drive and leave me there to get struck by some Boston driver. I knew he was completely frustrated, but he said nothing. He didn't even wheel me to Storrow Drive. Once on the road, after a few tense moments, he reached over for my hand. What a giant. Tom is truly a GIANT!! Thank God he understood that I had to protect our baby. Tom held my hand, squeezed it, and I knew he understood.

Today my boss, who is an Ophthalmologist, called from Hawaii. He's been on vacation and had only just heard about the cancer this afternoon. He told me something made him call the office despite his vacationing and the long distance. I briefed him about the whole CT scan and MRI controversy, and he asked me for the doctor's name and phone number at the Brigham. I am so very thankful I work for a doctor.

My boss actually paged this radiologist from the beaches of Hawaii to discuss my unique case. With that, the radiologist has called me from his conference meeting. I was able to speak directly to him and begin learning about this fancy MRI machine at the Brigham and Women's Hospital.

There's only one problem... I needed my doctor to order the biopsy. He explained, "You just can't walk in off the street or call and order your own tests and surgery. Why did you call me on your own like this anyway?" I replied that I would get the orders that he needed and that he would not believe me if I told him the story, but then proceeded to explain how I walked out of the first biopsy at the Mass General and about my mad search through the yellow pages. The radiologist was astonished.

March 30, 2000

There are many doctors who do not feel the biopsy can be done successfully through MRI. Evidently they feel that the radiologist will not be able to get a good enough picture. Actually, I have learned that several films or shots would be taken as the surgeon moved the needle into the proper location for sampling of the

Impossible Choices

lesion. The needle would also have to be guided back out again. I keep thinking of the radiation exposure during the CT scan. After speaking with the physician at Brigham, he needs my original MRI films to see the location of the lesions before determining if the biopsy can be done successfully. He also wants to see me because he needs to make sure that my stomach is not too large which would get in the way of the magnetic field. I am nineteen weeks pregnant and showing quite a mound, but I assured him that I am a tiny person and this would help.

I saw my new doctor friend this afternoon. It was then that I found out I would be making history at the Brigham, in all of Boston for that matter, because I was the first pregnant woman to have a surgical procedure in this machine. I also learned this machine is called MRT and not MRI. Magnetic resonance therapy as opposed to magnetic resonance imaging. Therapy meaning to actually treat as opposed to imaging to diagnose. That is the big difference with all the other regular MRI machines. This wonderful contraption is used to perform brain surgery. It is the only one of its kind in Boston. I feel lucky to have found it but I am quite frightened by the seriousness of it all.

This radiologist who would do the surgical bone biopsy finagled me into an operating room schedule tomorrow—Friday. This is just three days later than the CT scan biopsy at the Mass General. I am so grateful to him. I cried and cried. With reassurance, he said softly, "Oh, please don't cry. I'm going to help you." I am exhausted by my efforts, I hope he is right.

I met with him and another radiologist for one hour, and they believe the biopsy can be done and my belly will fit inside the machine. Following our meeting, a wonderful medical secretary Pam helped me prepare for tomorrow's procedure. I so desperately needed someone to coordinate my care because I was completely exhausted from all the footwork I had been doing. No one told me to seek medical advice elsewhere. I have done this on my own because there is so much at stake. I feel this is something I need to do.

I was sent for preoperative blood-work and an EKG. After that, I saw a high risk OB/GYN there at the Brigham and Woman's Hospital who discussed my case at great length. Again I was given hope for my unborn baby. The obstetrician spent a long time consulting with me about the whole cancer and chemotherapy issue relating to the baby. As well, we discussed the radiation risks and benefits from the diagnostic testing. She agreed with me about my concerns that I would no doubt need more testing if the biopsy was positive for cancer, and that each test would accumulate rads of radiation to the baby. This lovely doctor was so sensitive to my situation and offered me more hope. Moreover, she commended me in my unending efforts to protect my baby. After an eight hour day at the Brigham, I am ready for the MRT guided bone biopsy tomorrow at six o'clock in the morning.

Leaving the hospital, my eyes remained fixed on a woman in a wheelchair. She appeared to be waiting for a ride. I focused steadily on her bald head which revealed a half moon shaped scar held together with staples. She was pale and sad looking. Tom and Julie hurried past her, but I was compelled to stop. I reached out my hand to her and said, "You look like you could use a handshake, better yet a hug." My eyes filled with tears as we exchanged a warm greeting.

I told her of my own dilemma. She too had metastatic breast cancer which had gone to her brain. What if the cancer should go to my brain? Dear Lord, don't let that happen! We wished each

Impossible Choices

other luck; I tearfully hobbled away on my crutches. Once in the car, Julie apologized for not waiting, opting instead to rush straight to the car. She explained that she could not bear the sight of the patient with the horrific scar. My husband asked, "Why did you do that?" and I answered truthfully, "Because I wanted to."

April 1, 2000

It's Saturday. I am home now, recuperating from the surgical bone biopsy. Before the biopsy, I felt very well cared for, especially, with respect to the baby. The morning of the big event, the obstetrician had reviewed the procedure with regard to anesthesia and the risks to the baby. The biopsy would take two hours, so anesthesia was a concern. When I was asked if I had allergies and I answered, "No, but my husband does," three more anesthesiologists were called in. Wrong answer! Everything came to a screeching halt. The baby would have a fifty percent chance of having malignant hyperthermia which is an allergy to anesthesia—an anesthesiologist's nightmare. I was given an epidural instead of anesthesia and had to be awake through the entire procedure, which was absolutely unnerving. I was confined, strapped in, and on my side for three and half hours.

At one point, I counted nine people in the operating room. (You would have thought I was having that brain surgery) The anesthesiologist and the nurses did their best to keep me calm by occasionally talking to me, but they were very busy doing whatever they were supposed to be doing. Once inside the tube, my body was mostly emerged, and I was unable to see faces. They would reach their hand inside and stroke my head telling me what a great job I was doing.

I was terrified, and remaining calm was difficult. The noises around me were unpleasant, especially the sound of the hammering of my bone. Two surgeons worked skillfully as they spoke in hushed, serious tones. I could not hear their words because sounds were muffled in the tube. I did hear a grunt or two from the surgeon who was trying to get a sample of my bone that contained the tumor. It was vital that he obtain an adequate specimen in order for the biopsy to be successful.

The procedure seemed to be taking forever and I was growing more and more anxious. My poor little baby. My face was so close to the sides of the machine that I asked to have the pillow removed from beneath my head to give me space to exhale. I was listening to that hammering, *THA-DA-THA-DA-THA-DA-THA-DA...*

I could feel pressure, not pain, from the surgeon trying to get that piece of bone free. I could tell he was working intensely. If I were an old woman, perhaps the bone would have been brittle and more willing to come free. But I am young. I am so young. Way too young for all of this. They had to use another type biopsy needle, which meant guiding back out then going back in. We were already at the predetermined two-hour mark with still no biopsy. The hammering began again, and it was grotesque, but it was better than a drill. I settled my nerves by having thoughts about the baby—good thoughts. I decided that I was not alone in that tube at all. My little one was right there with me.

At long last, a specimen was retrieved from my iliac wing. And yet another doctor was called into the operating room to review the sample. This was someone from cytology who would decide if there was enough tumor present for an exact pathology result to confirm cancer. Nope! They would have to go back in for another sample... we were now three hours into the procedure. I was beginning to feel tingling sensations in my feet and legs, when I

Impossible Choices

overheard the anesthesiologist tell the surgeons that the epidural was only effective for three hours. Pressure sensation was beginning to feel like pain, and I was wild with anxiety. The anesthesiologist came over to me and relayed to me that the surgeons would only need a half hour more. He explained that the epidural would still be mainly effective. If I felt too much pain, they could give me a shot for localized pain.

My anxiety left me feeling nauseous. I was given an oxygen mask. Additionally, my shoulder was in great discomfort from bearing all my weight for so long. Lest we forget that I was strapped to a metal grid and bound with duct tape to keep me perfectly still.

I moved my head ever so slightly; the oxygen mask slipped off my mouth and nose up over my eyes. Part of the plastic was covering my mouth and nose. I was panting for air and thought that I would surely suffocate. Meanwhile, the oxygen was flowing quite nicely right into my eyes, drying them out! In my panic it seemed like ten minutes before someone rescued me, (I'm sure it was less than sixty seconds). It was awful not to be able to use my own arms to rescue myself. This little ritual took place several more times.

After three and a half-hours, the biopsy was completed, and the doctors were all quite pleased that the procedure had been a success. I was pulled out of the MRT tube, and the two surgeons came right over and commended me for a job well done. They were remarkably thankful to me for being so "heroic," as they said. I reached for their hands, taking them into my own, saying, "Thank you, thank you so much." I did not feel so heroic inside. I was screaming and kicking. I just clutched their hands for a very long moment. We had done it together as a team, and there had been no radiation to the baby. The baby's heartbeat was being monitored and doing just fine, and there was no radiation exposure. I was relieved and felt the whole thing was worth my exertion because my baby was safe.

April 7, 2000

As predicted, the biopsy was positive for metastatic breast cancer. What a week of waiting it has been. Today, Tom and I met with my oncologist and the high risk obstetrician at Mass General about the course of treatment. The plan is to use low dose chemotherapy. They have chosen an agent which they have experience with in pregnancy. This particular chemotherapy consists of large molecules, and will not cross the placenta. The OB is confident that I can even carry the baby full term. However, my oncologist has warned me of the long and difficult road ahead. She explained how complex it will be to receive chemotherapy at the same time I was carrying the baby. My body is in for a hard work out. No problem! I would run a marathon, climb any mountain, do whatever it takes. Whatever it takes. I've been in training all my life for this moment.

I still need a few more tests to rule out the spread of the disease to my liver or lungs. Furthermore, the tumor sample they've just gotten will be stained and tested for a gene called HER2/neu. This HER2/neu tissue testing has been done, and is currently being done, ever since my original diagnosis in 1997. Twenty-five to thirty percent of women with breast cancer have tumors that are HER2/neu positive. Barring the results of any further findings, my oncologist is saying she is still not positive that I should keep the pregnancy. She is reluctant to advise until the remaining tests come back. She told me that since I am her patient, she has to think about me. It's clear she is distraught with the whole situation. She knows how much this baby was wanted. Over the past six months, she has received all the letters from physicians I consulted with about

Impossible Choices

becoming pregnant after breast cancer. She even remembers at our first meeting three years ago that we had discussed at length about a future pregnancy. Now she's crying right along with me.

At my last appointment she gave me a generous, heartfelt hug. I appreciate her compassion. How difficult it must be for her to have the double-edged burden of what's right for my baby is the worst thing for me, her patient. I am certain this has been a tremendous strain on her part. It seems that I have shaken the very stability of her practice in medicine. But she has held firm and steady, tightening her resolve to do what's best for me along the way.

As Tom and I walked out of her office today, I spotted a young woman with a turban. Obviously she had been in treatment. She also had the most adorable baby girl in her arms. I knew she must have had chemotherapy during her pregnancy because the baby appeared to be only a couple of months old. During the three years I have been going to the breast center, I have never seen a baby there. It appeared that this mother received chemotherapy, and her baby is just fine. Not just fine, she is beautiful! I believe it's a sign!

Although, I learned that the one big difference in our medical status is that she was just diagnosed for the first time while pregnant and the cancer has not spread. I on the other hand, have metastasized. This makes my prognosis a lot worse. I told her my own story, and we cried together. I'm going to save our baby! I'm not going to terminate this pregnancy! I can have the chemotherapy just as we researched before the pregnancy.

April 8, 2000

Today I called my boss Andy at his home to let him know that I wouldn't be back to work, that I would be going out on disability. Andy was speechless. His silence on the other end of the phone

Barbara Dooling

was choking me up. We said our good-byes, he wished me good luck, and stressed that if there was anything I needed, that I could count on him. I knew that I could. That was about it, he assured me that he would call soon.

I feel so empty and frightened. The family—both Tom's and mine—call non stop. Thank God no one has pressured us about the decision of whether or not to continue the pregnancy. Each of Tom's sisters—Margaret, Tricia, Carolyn and Donna—support us no matter what we do. There's been talk that they would all help Tom to raise Kara and the baby if I die. On the other hand, it seems that my family doesn't really want me to go through with the pregnancy. They don't want me to die.

Russ says nothing—absolutely nothing. He's quite good at hiding his feelings. I don't fault him. I know he loves me. Sometimes you just have to understand a person. Ann is the one who talks to me. She doesn't think I'm strong enough to endure the pregnancy and the cancer. She loves me like a sister and I'm sure she doesn't want to lose me. Kenny keeps crying. He calls… he cries… he calls… he cries. He's just like Dad with the crying, but I do love his sensitivity. Paul and Maureen call from Colorado. Paul feels helpless. He is in disbelief that I could die. He does not believe in abortion. He loves me. He now believes in abortion for certain circumstances. Mary is devastated. She does not want me to keep the baby. She doesn't say this but I know her like a book. She thinks the pregnancy will kill me. No, the cancer will kill me. Geno keeps his clan of four kids praying. I think he commands them every day: pray, pray, pray. He tells me the kids are all praying. The kids are praying day and night. Mom and Dad? Oh forget Mom and Dad. I lie half the time when I talk to them on the telephone. They have no clue what is going on. If they only knew that the doctors want me to

Impossible Choices

terminate the pregnancy, they would call the Pope.

April 9, 2000

I'm scheduled for this Monday to have X-rays of my right shoulder and femur, an X-ray of my lungs, and an MRI of my abdomen to check for metastasis in the liver. I will be shielded with a lead apron for the X-rays. I am out of my mind with worry about the radiation to the baby. As well, I will have a fetal ultrasound to determine the exact gestation of the baby and to look for any abnormalities. Tom and I have already seen the baby's head on the previous MRI films. He is wondering if I will be able to handle looking at the ultrasound since it will be more vivid and we will see the baby's heart beating. I told him I have already felt the baby move, and I've already heard the heartbeat with the Doppler machine. I refuse to think of terminating the pregnancy, and I want to see our baby. I have to stay strong; I just have to stay very, very strong.

This afternoon I was praying for a miracle at Mission Church in Boston. It was my first time in this particular house of worship. My friends Kim and Fran took me to a healing mass. Father McDonough, who is quite notable for his healing ministry, was to officiate the mass only he was hospitalized for an illness. Ah well, I still prayed. I prayed for strength. I prayed to the Blessed Mother to help me with my decision. I envisioned and clung to her sacred heart, for the Blessed Mother herself had suffered the loss of her son. She knew my pain. As I asked for her gracious guidance, I clutched my stomach. I painfully got down on my knees and knelt in front of the altar. I focused on the beautiful adornments around me. I praised Jesus and all my favorite saints. I prayed to the sacred heart of the Lord. His holiness had great suffering. I sent my plea to his sacred heart. Tears streamed down my cheeks dropping onto the bench in front of me. For a short while I felt sanctity, although I was not given any solutions. Perhaps the answers lay ahead; perhaps I was never to find out. I could not lose my faith now. I prayed for a miracle. The miracle I prayed for was to save my baby. It was not to save my life.

April 10, 2000

The fetal ultrasound revealed that our baby was moving and appears to be healthy. Though we originally did not want to find out the sex of the baby, at this point, we asked the technician. She showed us all the body parts including the genitals. The female genitals... Our baby's a girl! I laughed and cried, and cried some more. I'm so excited that Kara will have a sister! I'm thinking of all the adorable clothes Kara has that I will be able to use again. What joy! This news brings me the strength I need.

We were given the usual pictures of the baby from the ultrasound, and Tom wheeled me out of the doctor's office. I just reached back and held on to my husband with one hand, and with the other, I held the angel pin that was fastened to my sweater. I've worn the angel every day. Mary gave me the pin when I found out I was pregnant. It's like a guardian angel for our baby. I never go out of the house without my little angel pin. I can't think about the cancer. I won't think about the cancer. It's been a wonderful day.

This evening I'm laying on the couch trying to alleviate the pain with ice packs strategically placed on top of my thigh, underneath my leg and behind my back. Family, friends and neighbors come and go. So many have visited me tonight. I showed them the five ultrasound pictures: a little foot with tiny toes, a front and side view of the head, the curved spine, and the little tiny hand.

Some folks choose not to see the pictures. These are the people

Impossible Choices

who have once rubbed my belly and have now stopped. I'm not angry with them. I have to understand. Even Tom has stopped feeling my stomach. At times I am so alone with this baby. Others can separate themselves so easily, but I cannot. The baby is in my body... growing... living. It is not so easy to detach myself; I am physically and emotionally affected. Tom goes back and forth with his decision. When he holds back his link to our baby, I am totally isolated. Again, I cannot be angry with him. In my heart I realize he is only thinking of me, his wife, and the mother of our three-year-old daughter. Tom is not prepared for any of this, especially to lose me. I understand him completely. He has doubts, and he's terrified of the consequences. I guess I am too, but I'm unwilling to give up. Please God, don't let us get ripped apart by this.

April 11, 2000

Test, tests, and more tests! I am losing my mind trying to keep the baby safe through all this diagnostic testing. I'm a worried mess; my nerves are shattered. The chest X-ray has revealed a small spot on my right lung, and another X-ray of my right shoulder shows cancer. My liver and other organs in the stomach area are clean. The tumor removed from the bone biopsy is positive for the HER2/neu gene. This means a more aggressive cancer, and it also means treatment with an antibody drug called Herceptin. The Herceptin is a laboratory manufactured protein that targets a very specific site on the surface of the breast cancer cell. I need the Herceptin to stop the overproduction of a certain protein my body produces. This drug, consisting of smaller molecules, WILL cross the placenta and cannot be given to me without potentially causing birth defects to the baby. I just can't believe it. I am horrified. This is a terrible blow.

I can't help but remember my friend Annmarie and how she

fought for her life. Her two children are now living without their mother. My heart aches for Kara. I recall that Annmarie's cancer, like mine, was also positive for HER2/neu. The cancer had circulated her body like quicksand. She died waiting for the drug Herceptin which was not yet on the market. This antibody had only been used in clinical trial studies; you had to be chosen in a lottery to receive the drug. Annmarie died in September of 1998 and the drug came out for use on the general public in November of 1998. Now this Herceptin is at my immediate disposal, while Annmarie died waiting for it.

April 12, 2000

Another call from yet another doctor, confirming that the cancer is aggressive and spreading rapidly. I need to begin treatment immediately... or else! How insane is this situation? If I begin treatment immediately, my baby will be damaged, perhaps fatally. And if I postpone treatment, I may die waiting for treatment like Annmarie.

I am sitting on the front porch as the sun goes down on this beautiful spring day. How can things be so wrong on such a pleasant day? We know that the biopsy I just had on the left pelvic region is cancer. In addition to this, an X-ray of the right leg and hip, which is where my pain originated, has a very large tumor. I'm in so much pain that I haven't been able to sleep. I'm afraid to take the prescribed narcotics because of the baby. I continue my icing and crawling. With this new information, the orthopedic oncologist will perform a surgical procedure called open reduction with internal fixation by inserting three screws to secure the femur and prevent fracturing. I am terrified the baby won't survive the operation. Forever concerned for Jenna Rose. Our baby now has a name.

Impossible Choices

I have a few days to wait for the surgery. I am going to one more specialist tonight. Kim has given me the name of a Perinatologist at Beth Israel Hospital. He is a high risk OB particularly with premature births. I want to see about delivering the baby early.

I'm home now, safely tucked into my bed. What a physical and emotional wreck, I am! The evening was so agonizing that I got sick to my stomach and vomited profusely outside the hospital. I threw up all over myself. My hands were shaking, and I began to cry uncontrollably. Once inside, the first minutes during the office visit, I just sobbed. I knew that I must calm myself down in order to have a productive consultation. It was vital that I obtain the most advice that I possibly could.

Tonight I learned the baby would not survive if delivered today, and I might not survive if I wait until a safer month for the baby. Additionally, the risk of birth defects is seventy-six percent up to twenty-seven weeks gestation—that's almost ten weeks away! But it is not the birth defects that I am worried about, because I could live with a child with birth defects. The problem is that it is likely that neither of us would survive the ordeal if we waited a month or two. She would still be too young to be successfully delivered. We have an inversely related survival situation happening. I am going to throw up again. I just can't endure this.

Each day that passes, I continue to bond with my Jenna Rose as she moves about inside me. The doctor was so kind and sympathetic to our situation. Despite the deplorable conversation, this doctor delivered his information with such compassion. He had an extraordinary manner in which he conveyed his expertise. But really, he could not help us.

Barbara Dooling

April 13, 2000
I attended my support group this evening where the women formed a circle around me in solidarity. We held hands with a firm grip, each of them giving me a strong hug. We all cried together.

One of the other members, Ellen, is also pregnant. I can only imagine how frightened she is to learn that I was diagnosed with the cancer spreading. Ellen and I are about two weeks apart in our pregnancies. But she has had no problems and is doing beautifully. I don't understand how our conditions can be so very different. Cancer certainly is a cruel and unpredictable demon. Over the past couple of years, Ellen and I have shared the same anguish and worries about getting pregnant after breast cancer. I remember her saying to me, "You've got to live your life." So after years of talking about it and dreaming about it, we're both pregnant. So what happened? Why did my pregnancy go so awry? I am obviously very happy for her, I just don't understand why things couldn't have worked out equally as well for me... Why God? Please tell me why. Won't you give me a sign, God? I really need to hear from You right now.

Ellen and I had planned to walk the relay for life together. This relay is a fund raiser for cancer research. It is held in cities all across the United States. Our local relay is to be held at the high school track and field. Some of the women in our group formed a team to participate in the relay. We call ourselves the Earth Angels. We are planning to have tee-shirts made with our team name printed on the back. Part of the celebration will include a survivor's lap in which all cancer survivors walk around the track. Just like last year, at dusk, luminary bags which line the entire track, will be lit in memory of those who have died of cancer, and for those who are still fighting the battle. Everyone knew how much it meant that

Impossible Choices

Ellen and I team up for the survivor's lap. And now I wonder if I will ever fulfill our quest.

April 14, 2000

I think about my pregnancy with Kara. It was a joyous time. I loved being pregnant. I loved the way I looked. I felt radiant and remarkably healthy. I love being pregnant this time too. I want this baby for Kara, for Tom, and for me. I cannot consent to terminate the pregnancy, and I'm told the procedure must be done within one more week.

The procedure has now been explained to me; I am even more horrified. The OB/GYN at Mass General defined a method, which I could not fathom. I was told I could not be put to sleep because the birthing process would take too long. I would also be on the regular maternity floor, therefore I would hear other woman giving birth or babies crying. Worst of all, I am having nightmares that the baby will still be alive after it comes out. How would I survive this? I think surely that I would have a nervous break down if I were to have to end my baby's life and push her out of my body. I am sickened. Sickened. Why? I will never understand, God, why this is happening.

The doctors are suggesting that I have the surgery to secure my hip and femur bone first so that my femur and hip won't fracture pushing the baby out. Then two days later would be the fetal ablation. I want to get on a plane and escape far away. I told Tom I would not come back until it was too late to take the baby. I am a nervous wreck and cry constantly. The stress has made me nauseous and I am vomiting several times a day. When I am finally able to force food into my mouth, I can't keep it down.

Tom was sorrowful when I told him that we should just have

the baby and who cares if I die. His eyes were glassy, and he looked so distressed. He said that Kara needed me and so did he. He reminded me that the baby might not even make it to thirty-two weeks, and then everyone would be dead, and what was the point of that? I cursed the cancer that had invaded my body! I cursed and I cursed!

April 17, 2000
  I agreed to terminate the pregnancy. I was numb—completely and utterly devastated, both in body and spirit. Had I done my absolute best to find a better solution than this one? God knows that I had. Then, God, please tell me why trying our best doesn't always bring success? I need to know why. Please send me a sign to let me know that I'm doing what You want me to do. I can live with that. As long as I know that I am doing what you want I will be able to survive this. I beg you to send me a sign.
  Mary brought the folks to our home where I broke down crying while attempting to explain everything. I began to deliver the news, but I could not finish. Tom and my sister had to explain. I sat bawling and trembling. They took it like real troopers. After being married for fifty-five years and raising six children, they've had their share of shocking news. They tried to be strong for my sake, but I could read their faces. And their silence only meant they were afraid to speak. Dad's eyes filled with tears. Mom was dazed, staring down at the floor. I felt her pain. She was after all, grieving for her own baby—me.
  Tom and I lay in bed that evening embracing one another. For the first time in three weeks, he touched my stomach. He held my belly; his hands were warm and soothing. He felt our baby move. We lay in silence... there was nothing more to say. There was nothing

Impossible Choices

more to do. We were both exhausted. We clung to each other with great fear of the days ahead. We were definitely in the eye of the storm and I wondered if we would ever reach the safe harbor. I believe that Tom wondered if I would ever be the same again. I definitely would not ever be the same. I feared losing my mind. I thought about people who lived through the holocaust. Why was I preoccupied with such horror? I thought about how any of those people could have survived. What kept some of them alive during the vicious torture? How could they go on living after watching their loved ones killed? What allowed them to persevere? Where did their courage come from? How did those who did survive go on living with such horror imbedded in their heads? I wondered if my conscience could live after my own horror was over. I wondered if my heart would turn to stone. Sleep did not come at all this night.

April 21, 2000

I awoke from the surgery which secured my femur and hip in an active recovery ward full of fellow patients. Nurses were dashing with fervor, making their rounds. I was crying and pleading for someone to check the baby's heartbeat. I kept repeating myself to anyone who neared my bed. I persisted with my plea, "Is my baby all right? Please, someone tell me if my baby is okay? Will someone help me to see if my baby's heart is still beating?" I was frantic. I was still trying to protect her. I was in a great deal of pain and given morphine for relief. The effects of the drug finally put me to sleep.

The next time I woke up, I was in my own room dizzy and vomiting. I spewed all day and throughout the night. There was nothing left but I continued with dry heaves, which lasted for three whole days. Tom never left my side. He nursed me, including emptying the bedpan and washing my body with warm face cloths. I became so

Barbara Dooling

weak that I could scarcely lift my head or move. Like the sentinel, Tom kept a watchful eye on me night and day. He dozed for brief periods on a cot next to my bed. I am grateful to have such a genuine man at my side. He held my hand and whispered into my ear the pledge he made on our wedding day, repeating over and over; "In sickness and in health, I love you forever, in sickness and in health." I worried for his own health as I began to see that the stress was taking its toll on him. Dark circles smudged the skin underneath his eyes… still he kept his vigil.

I lay there thinking how my perfect world was falling apart. The earth was quaking below me; I was being swallowed by a giant crack in the ground. But Tom was there, pulling me back safely. His grip is so gentle and soothing. I thought about how we had struggled and agonized about the fate of our unborn child. Our hearts were ripped apart by the decision, yet Tom never uttered an unkind word or raised his voice to me. He remained by my side, emotionally and physically my teammate. He is my very best friend—forever.

My hematocrit level, the red blood cells which carry oxygen, was low. I had two blood transfusions which were ordered by the orthopedic oncologist. Because of this unexpected complication, my hospital stay went from overnight to eight days. Once my condition was stabilized, I would be moved to another hospital for the therapeutic termination of my pregnancy.

We waited anxiously for the abnormal blood levels to regulate. Each morning the orthopedic oncologist and his team of residents visited my bedside. I suspect the residents were getting quite an education with my complicated medical case. They all conducted themselves cautiously and were rather shy whenever they approached. My orthopedic surgeon was one of the best. I learned

Impossible Choices

he had pioneered many a procedure at this hospital over the years. Despite his years, his skills were trustworthy, and I could tell by his firm handshakes and even his gripping hugs that his hands were still steady.

It was evident that his skills not only involved manipulating bones and using a scalpel, but over his many seasons, he had also acquired a sparkling bedside manner. He was jovial, warm, and comical. He was full of hope, and this gave me hope. However, my pregnant stomach and the knowledge of what lay ahead for me disturbed him. He was brought to tears at my bedside as he held my hand and spoke to me. I hoped the resident doctors, who shadowed him daily, memorized his actions and his words. I hoped they embedded this vision in their minds for all their own future patients.

This fine doctor took my hands and tightly held them in his own. With a firm, steady gaze, he looked me in the eyes and told me there was hope. He said that he was going to keep me alive, and he and I would dance together at Kara's wedding. I needed to hear those words of hope so very much. They were lifesaving words.

April 22, 2000

While I recovered, Tom had the task of staying in touch with the OB/GYN, updating him and postponing the next procedure twice. At one point this surgery to terminate the pregnancy was rescheduled for today, my birthday. All who knew us seemed uncomfortable about this and felt sorry for me. I, on the other hand didn't really mind. In fact, I thought it somewhat symbolic and wanted to share my birthday with our baby, Jenna Rose. But it was postponed just the same.

As it turns out, I am still too ill to be discharged. I have had no visitors except Tom and the stream of doctors and nurses who care for me. Thus, today, some friends and relatives visited with cake and ice cream, bringing gifts and well-intentioned conversation. Among them was my little girl, Kara Elizabeth. How joyous it was to see her after this long separation. Until this day, I had only spoken to her by telephone. We chatted and blew kisses and I tucked her in over the phone every night. She would innocently ask, "Mommy, when can I come home? Why you still in the hospital? I need you, Mommy! I need you!"

I assured my child, "Soon, my precious. Mommy will be home soon and we'll all be together again." As she revealed to me how much she missed me and needed me, I fought back the tears. Here was the justification for our plan of terminating the pregnancy. My daughter, Kara did need me. She did need her mother. Alive. By this point it was fairly certain that if the pregnancy continued, the cancer would speed to my brain and I would not survive. Even without terminating the pregnancy, the baby might not live either.

I am thirty-nine today. With my hospital room crowded from those who came to bring birthday wishes, Kara dashed to my bedside and hurled her small self up onto my lap. She leaped with such a vault that the bed rolled slightly. As I embraced my girly-girl, my eyes brimmed. I fluttered my eyelids to restrain the flow. Her first words were not hello. She curiously asked, "Mommy, is our baby okay? Is baby Jenna Rose still in your belly?" Her hands pulled open my hospital gown, and she examined my stomach. The group of birthday well-wishers were witness to this three year old girl's interrogation.

I was not expecting the question, but responded honestly by nodding yes. Up to this point, we had not told Kara much, only that Mommy was going into the hospital to have an operation to fix her

Impossible Choices

leg. How Kara drew her own conclusions, is anyone's guess. As they say, children absorb everything. As careful as we tried to be, it was evident she had heard something. Kara had been staying with her grandparents, and I suppose she heard conversation there as well. I shall spend the remaining days in the hospital trying to seek council on how to explain to Kara that she is not going to be a big sister. There is not going to be a baby.

April 23, 2000

Easter Sunday concluded this heart-wrenching weekend. Tom and I shared hospital food and held hands. There was no ham, no leg of lamb, no colored Easter eggs, no chocolate bunnies, and no Sunday mass with children dressed in fancy spring attire. Kara would not wear her pastel dress with shiny white Mary Janes and her flowered Easter bonnet. I had asked Grammy and Grampy not to mention the Easter Bunny, hoping we'd be able to have our own celebration when Mommy, Daddy, and Kara returned home. There were eggs to color, carrots and lettuce to leave for cottontail bunny, a basket to fill, and plastic eggs with hidden treats to find. Yes, we would have our Easter, and Kara was young enough that we could switch the real day without her realizing.

On this holy day, besides the festivities, I thought about something Tom's uncle Howard had said to us shortly before I went into the hospital. When he heard the news about the cancer spreading and the fetal ablation, he came to our home to give us a special blessing. We lit a candle and prayed together. As we gripped one another's hands, Uncle Howard compared our plight to that of Jesus' suffering on the cross on Good Friday. He told Tom and I that we were about to endure our own pain and suffering during the holy season. I believe his analogy.

Barbara Dooling

April 25, 2000

New hospital. Such a horrifying moment. We had an appointment at eleven o'clock to meet the doctor and begin the process of an abortion. Tom did not want me using the word. I hate the word myself. In fact, I despise that word. Abortion implies choice. Do I really have a choice? My choice is so obvious. My choice is to give birth to my miracle daughter. But that is not what is about to happen. This is not my choice. This is not an abortion. God knows my heart. God knows my circumstances. God knows that this is not my choice. The whole world can judge me wrongly if they choose. I only care about what God thinks. God knows. God will take my baby angel back home and tuck her safely in the palm of his hand.

As Tom and I entered the hospital, he somberly pushed me in my wheelchair down the corridor. Painfully I witnessed a couple with their newborn baby gliding blissfully through the main entrance. The new mother, too, was in a wheel chair. On top of her, nearly blocking her whole body, was the baby tucked inside an infant car seat. He or she was snugly wrapped in blankets and only its tiny red face was showing. The dad was pushing his family with one arm while managing a large black duffel strapped to his shoulder. In his other hand, he was carrying a small potted plant which had a balloon sailing above, bopping to and fro.

I forced a smile. It was as artificial as the silk plants and trees that lined the lobby. In my heart I was happy for them; there is no joy like that particular joy. But the contrast of their moment versus my moment was too great for me to bear. My heart was being yanked from my chest. Is there any other circumstance in the world that can compare to this? "Pulling the plug" perhaps, but not quite. Surely there is no other situation like this. Please don't judge me, my

Impossible Choices

heart screams to the world as we proceed down the hall. Come sit where I am sitting and show me what you would do.

Further on, we happened upon a table set up with a display of pamphlets and literature. Behind the exhibit was a cheerful, attractive woman, stylishly dressed. I beckoned for Tom to stop because the poster board sign read something about spiritual needs. If there was something I needed today, it was inspiration and spiritual support.

The lovely woman was the hospital chaplain. As it turns out after speaking to her about the pending procedure, she's going to help guide us through our dismal journey. She will make herself available to us for council throughout my stay.

April 27, 2000

The morning of the procedure, the chaplain held my hand at the very early hour of seven. Once I was whisked away into the operating room, she sat with Tom until she baptized our Jenna Rose. I am not sure if we would automatically have been referred had we not run into her in the lobby. Whatever the case, we greatly needed her. She was a comfort.

It is pouring rain outside, as it has been for several days. There has not been a ray of sunshine. It suites my dismal mood. All those long days as I lay in the hospital bed after the surgery to my leg, Tom and I talked to each other calmly and quietly. The TV in my room was never turned on and I had very few visitors. We just passed the hours loving each other. When there was nothing to say, we sat in silence, but the hush was not awkward for us. We seemed to comfort each other even in quiet. We were perfectly at ease without speaking. The stillness was the same as we waited in an examining room just two days ago to meet the obstetrician gynecologist—

Barbara Dooling

another new doctor. Tom and I did not speak.

The physician entered the room, and I began to tremble. He introduced himself and offered a welcoming handshake to both of us. He was as gentle as he could be while he tried to explain the procedure. He pulled from my chart, a consent form. I was breathless and crying. My head felt so light; I was hyperventilating. The doctor handed me a pen and waited for my signature. Tom and the doctor both waited; all eyes fixed on that darn form. My hand was shaking so much that I could not hold the pen correctly. The ink never touched the paper. Instead, my tears blotted the form, dropping down as quick as the rain outside.

I looked up at the two men in the room, my husband and this doctor. I spoke with a quivering voice, "I cannot sign." Tom said nothing. I sobbed uncontrollably. The doctor excused himself and said he would give us more time; he would return in one hour.

I was in a complete panic. I kept repeating to Tom, "I cannot do it; I cannot do it!" Then I sent my pleas out to God... Please, God, rescue me from this moment. Please help me, God. Please make someone else sign this consent form. This is NOT my consent. The only thing I consent to is your Will, God. Not my will but yours be done... I prayed aloud. I anxiously rubbed my hands together, wringing my fingers wildly until they became red and raw. I covered my mouth to keep from screaming and to block the air from my lungs. My respiration was forced through my fingers, trying to escape. I bolted up and paced the short distance of the room. I prattled on and on—meaningless words. Tom watched in terror. He could not even bring himself to touch me. He stood there helplessly without expression. This decision involved a lot of people, but in the end, the final signature was mine.

I used a phone in the examining room to page at least five

Impossible Choices

physicians who had been involved with my case. One by one, the calls were returned. Each doctor had the same news, the same advice. They reiterated all the facts that I already knew. Nothing changed about my situation. There was no miracle coming here. I had to come to terms with this horror. If I postponed treatment until after the pregnancy, my life was in great danger. I kept asking myself, "What went so terribly wrong after we had researched this matter so thoroughly before getting pregnant?" No doctor ever mentioned terminating the pregnancy if the cancer recurred.

I do not blame anyone. We had at least five opinions. Though I fault no one, I now realize the limits of medicine. Medicine is not an exact science. I kept thinking I had something to fall back on because I was told chemotherapy could be administered to a pregnant woman. Truth of the matter was, chemotherapy could be given, but the drug Herceptin could not. This was the new antibody drug being used to treat metastatic breast cancer with tumors having over expression of HER2/neu. It was devastating to find out about it now. I was plagued by "what ifs." What if I had had a bone scan before getting pregnant. What if I had had the HER2/neu test, what if, what if, what if! It was just not routinely done! It was far too late now.

The doctor came back precisely one hour later. Tom and I were grief stricken and frightened. I signed the consent form. An uncomfortable but brief procedure was done to open my cervix. As I understood the concept, laminaria twigs, which were tiny sticks made from seaweed, were inserted to stretch open the cervix. This would take twenty-four hours. Once in place, there was no turning back. I could not believe that I allowed the procedure. I was just numb.

I began cramping right away. I was admitted into the hospital.

Barbara Dooling

Then, it was over. Our baby, my baby was gone. No words could possibly console me. I was frightened that I'd become demented with grief. All my efforts to save the baby were futile. It was really over. After the procedure, I woke screaming with excruciating pain in my groin and hip. Nurses were trying to decipher the problem. I could see Tom leaning against a wall. His face was gray with fear. He kept asking the doctors if my hip had fractured during the procedure. Mary was also present. Her hands were tightly covering her mouth for fear she would let out a scream herself. She had tears in her eyes and I saw her flee the room. My shrieking continued.

I had never experienced such pain. I thanked God for this acute pain in my groin. I was grateful because I did not have to think about my baby Jenna Rose. The pain was piercing, shooting through worse than any spasm. I let out more shrieks with the slightest movement. I too thought my hip had fractured. Suddenly, I was whisked away to have an X-ray to rule out this possibility. I was given something for the pain and slipped into unconsciousness. And when I woke…

In the early dawn, as I opened my eyes, I met Tom's vigilant gaze. He was sitting beside me holding my hand. His face was weary and he looked so forlorn. His green eyes peered into my soul. We did not speak to one another. Outside the hospital window, rain continued to fall very hard. The downpour was loud during the silence. We both just listened to the precipitation. I was afraid to speak and I suspect so was Tom. I was depleted of all energy, both physically and mentally. I had a hollow feeling inside, churning in my stomach.

This was the pain I feared most—not the cancer pain, not the surgery pain, but the emotional pain. It was far worse. I grieved for

Impossible Choices

our baby. We grieved. How great was our sorrow! I was tormented with more "What ifs." I was in disbelief. I couldn't even cry because I feared that a nervous breakdown was surely coming, and I needed to stay strong. I could not lose my sanity. I had to fight for my life so that my daughter, Kara Elizabeth would have her mother. I could not collapse or break. I was silent. And Tom was silent. And the rain outside beat against the windows.

As the empty hours passed, I decided to write a eulogy for our baby.

The words came to mind rapidly. I knew just what I wanted to say. I scribbled my thoughts down and as I wrote, I quietly wept. My words were blurred on the page before me. The tears streamed. They were warm against my cheeks, and I allowed them to fall without stopping. It was no use wiping them away. I kept writing and I fought those tears until I became dizzy from holding my breath, but I kept writing. My nose was stinging, and my head was stuffed up. Finally, my tribute was complete. A good-bye letter to a baby I would never hold. If I could remove my heart from behind my ribs and rip it from my body, I would, for it was truly broken. I had never felt such sadness in all my life.

Tom handled all the burial arrangements from the hospital. Our baby daughter will be laid to rest at a cemetery in a section called "Angel Hill." Only babies are buried there. Ironically Tom and I have walked past this hill many times. I would stop to read the headstones and admire the collection of toys and stuffed animals on the graves. I did not know a single child who lay there, but I never passed it without crying. Tom would ask me why I tormented myself so, why I stopped when I knew very well it would upset me. Perhaps God was preparing me for the day that I would lay my own baby to rest in this bittersweet place. Yes, I believe it was a prepa-

Barbara Dooling

ration for future visits at "Angel Hill."

April 28, 2000

Cold and rainy. I've been discharged and began radiation and chemotherapy treatments immediately. The baby was buried. My family was sympathetic that I had to go into Boston to start treatment the same day we lay our Jenna Rose to rest. However, I am glad to be preoccupied. Our immediate family and close friends attended the service. There was no formal funeral, but we did have a service at the cemetery.

I have never been to a child's burial, and I was so moved to see such a tiny coffin. Tom had purchased a small cross of pink baby tea roses which was draped over the white casket. "Our little angel" was written on a pink and white bow. To one side stood a beautiful heart shaped arrangement that surrounded the tiny casket; it was made of pink roses and other assorted pink flowers. Our local funeral home had set up a tent and chairs. They never charged us for administering any of the various services, not even for the cost of the casket. This kind gesture was so much more than just charity.

Today is typical for early spring. Though it finally stopped raining, the air was damp and raw. I was shivering and resting my body against Tom. Our parents sat beside us. We all held hands firmly, as if to empower each other with strength. I was surprisingly calm. Though several of my doctors had offered different tranquilizers, I never took anything. I feared I would not be coherent and I wanted to remember the service.

Everything was peaceful. The flowers were so lovely, the casket pure white. The other headstones had remnants of Easter with stuffed bunnies and lilies adorning them. Uncle Howard read from

Impossible Choices

the bible and asked Sheila and Bruce—the godparents—to anoint the casket with holy water for a baptism. My eulogy for Jenna Rose was read aloud along with a thank you letter I had prepared for Tom and our family and friends. Afterward, we listened to a CD with the song *No More Tears in Heaven* written and recorded by Eric Clapton for his own young son who had died tragically. It is a sad yet comforting song. At the end of the song, two white doves were released into the air. They hovered overhead until they landed in a nearby tree. How lovely and peaceful was their delicate flight. I was amazed that they stayed in the tree. The birds were a gift from Russ and Ann. It was a most beautiful and tranquil closure.

April 29, 2000

One day has passed since we buried our Jenna Rose. I was gazing out the kitchen window this afternoon—my thoughts heavy and clouded, tears still dripping down my cheeks into the dish water—when all of a sudden a rainbow appeared from a sun shower sky! I quickly grabbed the camera to capture this miracle. Then I called Mom. With great wisdom and faith, she told me that Jenna Rose sent me this rainbow to tell me that everything was going to be all right. My sign from heaven!

After so much reflection these past forty-eight hours, a tiny ray of hope began to poke its way into my troubled thoughts. Perhaps God with his infinite wisdom and understanding searches our hearts for the motives and reasons behind our actions and choices, rather than judge us purely on the actions alone. Yes, surely my glorious God whom I have so faithfully worshipped and obeyed would do that. I slowly unlocked my clamped heart and allowed the rainbow to fill and heal my soul, and awaken my traumatized spirit. Thank you, God, for sending me a sign. Thank you, God, for your

Barbara Dooling

amazing love.

Tom and I brought Kara to Angel Hill, the section of the cemetery where children are buried, to tell her about Jenna Rose. As soon as we got out of the car and headed for the grave, I began to cry. I couldn't hold back the tears. All the pink flowers lay in a mound on the fresh grave. Tom spoke to Kara in a soft voice and told her our baby Jenna Rose was going to stay here with some other babies. He said that God was going to take care of her. She would live in heaven and not with us.

Kara immediately shouted, "You mean I not going to be a big sister? It's not fair! I want my baby!" I was shocked at her alert interpretation. Kara asked to see our baby. She cried, "I just want to see her and touch her. Just once, Mommy. Please go and get her so I can touch her just once. I promise, I'll let her go back to God." My heart ached for Kara. We had brought one single white rose for Kara to place on her sister's grave. With her small hand, she gripped that flower and gently tossed it among the heap. We did not linger. We did not want to magnify the moment.

May 12, 2000

It's been two weeks since the burial and I have finally begun to think about my own mortality. The reality has set in and I am now terrified about the fact that the cancer has returned. Before this moment, I had not fully grappled with the issue of the cancer having metastasized. My focus had been on the pregnancy—my precious Jenna Rose. Tonight, on this rainy evening, I am feeling so frightened. I actually have stage four breast cancer—and there is no stage five. Statistically, I am considered terminal. But I cannot think this way. I have to live for Kara and Tom. I must be here for my

Impossible Choices

beautiful family. I must find a way to live beyond "terminal."

I am horrified at what has transpired. No one, not Tom, nor the doctors, or my family knows the depth of my grief. It is deep within my soul... deeper than the fathoms of the ocean floor and as far as the universe reaches. I have tried to drive away these thoughts, but they haunt me. I am still bleeding from the termination of the pregnancy. It is a daily reminder of something I cannot ever reverse. Each time I go to the bathroom, dress myself, or bathe, I am haunted. My mind seems to play tricks on me. At times, I can still feel movement. The feeling is like little nudges, not gas. I wonder... am I going crazy?

I am so distraught. I was compelled to go to the grave tonight to beg for Jenna Rose's help. I wanted to plead with her to take care of me so that Kara will grow up with her mother. I had to tell Jenna Rose how frightened I am of the cancer. I have begun to think of Jenna Rose as my contact in heaven. She is very real to me, my suffering with Jenna Rose is very real, which now makes heaven very real to me. It seems as though maybe that's why God sent us Jenna Rose. He wanted me to have a real angel. Maybe God knew I would need a real angel to get me through this next phase of my life—stage IV cancer. Well... it worked God! I just want you to know that Your plan worked. My angel of trauma is helping me with my trauma right now. Thank you, God. I am proof that having a real angel makes heaven more real and You more real, God. What I mean by real angel is one who comes down from heaven and touches us physically, then returns to heaven, leaving a chord to heaven. Jenna Rose kissed the palm of my hand, and now I can feel that God is keeping her, and me, safe in the palm of His hand through my trauma. My body can feel this as well as my heart. Yep, I can feel this physically now, whereas I never could before Jenna Rose came into our lives. God, I hope you won't mind some venting. I really need to vent tonight.

It was after eight in the evening and the cemetery was deserted. Who would have the poor sense to be visiting a grave this late at night in the cold rain? I dropped my crutches and knelt on the delicate new grass which has begun to sprout on top of the freshly dug grave. There is still no headstone. The grave is bare except for the few trinkets Kara has left on a previous visit. There in the pouring rain, I prayed. I began to sob. Clenching my fists, I thrust them into the muddy ground. I pounded the wet dirt over and over and over again until I was weak. My words and sobs turned into screams. I lost all control. I screeched until the shrills of my voice became hoarse—my throat dry and coarse. My leg was piercing with pain; my fists throbbed. My clothes were completely drenched. I lifted myself off the ground, wondering if anyone in the neighborhood had heard the commotion. Surely they would have thought someone was being murdered. The tender young grass was crushed and flattened. My thoughts settled there for an extra moment. The grass would recover and so would I. I collected myself and drove home shaking from the cold and tremendous screaming. I needed that good cry, and I needed to communicate with my Jenna Rose.

May 13, 2000

More encouraging cards from everyone—friends, cousins, and even the nieces and nephews! As we approach Mother's Day, I'm going to need them! Ann continues with meals-on-wheels for us. Uncle Lawrence and Aunt Phyllis, Mom and Dad Dooling and Mom and Dad gave us a generous amount of money; it will all help with many expenses like buying a headstone for Jenna Rose, parking at

Impossible Choices

the hospital, and insurance copayments! Andy sent more lovely flowers. He's such a gem. Kenny calls every week; Mary still calls daily! Geno and the kids make tiny crosses out of palms for Jenna's grave. Uncle Howard and Aunt Jackie visit and pray with us. Everyone has been so kind. Their abiding love and prayers have been sincere. This is what sees us through each day. We are grateful for the constant, steadfast support. Indeed, we continue to endure this suffering by drawing strength and stability from our family and friends. They endow us with stamina and courage. We are still stunned by the heavy blows, but we are confident that we shall get through these dark days with the help of so many wonderful people. We know how much they love us! We believe in them!

My days are never too long as I fight this battle. I am tolerating the weekly treatments extremely well with the exception of some fatigue. I am thankful since I am in it for the duration—until there is a cure. My prognosis is frightening, however, I have a special little girl counting on me so I must not give up. Kara and Tom are recovering, too. We all seem to have slipped back into a routine and this helps Kara feel more stable. She had a bit of difficulty adjusting when I first came home from the hospital. During the nights she would cry out for me. I would hold her tightly but she feared that I was going to leave her. We let her sleep in the big bed with us for a few nights and she loved this. She had also wet her pants a couple of times. It was more upsetting for her since Kara has been potty trained since she was two years old. We did not make anything of it and the problem was short lived. We are fortunate that Kara has regained her confidence as she realizes that Mommy isn't going anywhere, and we are all a family again.

How difficult it is to be a statistic, especially when you want to prove them wrong. My spirits are exceptionally good, considering what has happened. I owe that to family and friends who continue to support me with their unending love and prayers. Despite this dreadful disease, I am still smiling. I love my husband and small daughter, and I love my simple life. I can't look back on the tragedy. I must live with what I have, all of which is great, and not cease to live fully because of what I do not have. I do believe with all my heart that I have every reason to live happily.

I will try to stay positive and keep pushing forward. I have lost a very big battle and the wounds have left deep scars. The scars that are on my body are not nearly as branded as the ones that linger in my head. Though the battle may have been lost, I shall keep fighting to win the war. This soldier, this warrior may still struggle in combat to pull off a victory! I will heal my mind with time and love. The love which surrounds me is my healing power—my restoration.

May 14, 2000
It is a happy Mother's Day despite my great loss of Jenna Rose. I am happy and so grateful for my Kara. Today I think about my own mother... I was wondering how she decided to name me after her. It's not too often a baby girl gets named after her mother. I'm not complaining here, on the contrary, I rather like the idea. I'm proud to be her little junior.

When Tom and I heard that I was pregnant for the second time with another girl, I wanted to name the baby Rose. Like a rose that returns every spring, I was feeling renewed in my health. Having been diagnosed with breast cancer after Kara was born, I prayed to God to save my life so she would have her mommy. Then the news of my recent pregnancy gave me new hope. The thorns upon a rose were the cancer, but the lovely flower was my baby girl.

Impossible Choices

My mom taught me that sometimes life does have sharp thorns. However, with their sharpness comes beauty. I am saddened that Jenna Rose did not live to hear her pretty name spoken. It is quite moving that our baby's due date was in August on my mom's birthday, and she died just four days after mine. The baby shares our birthdays.

And now that the cancer is back, I pray once more for God's mercy so Kara will grow up with the love of her mother. Although my own mother had a chemical imbalance which nearly destroyed her, she had an invincible spirit. Yes, she had a lion's courage to raise six children during toilsome years. I have wonderful memories of her unyielding love. I feel blessed to have had her all my life. It leaves me with great pain to think my daughter would be robbed of knowing her own mother. Part of who I am today is Mom. From her I have learned about maternal love, which is one of the strongest unconditional loves. She taught me about family love which is one of the strongest bonds. As well, she showed me the value of marital love which is one of the strongest commitments. Mom guided me through spiritual love which is divine and whole. And she educated me about self identity which is love and respect for one's self. Collectively, these values are part of the very person she prepared me to be.

Thank you, Mom. I love you.

May 25, 2000

I set myself on autopilot for doctors' appointments, cancer treatments, and diagnostic tests. I just do what I have to do. I try to block the ugly part of these days and lift my mind to a happier place while going through the motions. What a constant struggle it is. I know that I must have courage and faith. Tom and our little Kara are

Barbara Dooling

the reasons I keep fighting. I cannot let myself become depressed or angry. It is time to move on. Though it is difficult, I try not to spend my time wondering about the future. After all, the future is a big mystery. It is a surprise. I must acknowledge that the past is over and the present is right now. I love now. I wake up every morning, so thrilled to have another morning. Despite this dreadful disease which has stolen so much already, I must be grateful for what I have. I cannot go back to those depressing days in March and April. I must not take myself to those horrid moments. I shall go forward and heal physically and emotionally. I must! Bitterness is hateful and ugly and does not wear well on any person. I shall not let my daughter see that happen to her mother. She, Kara Elizabeth, is my medicine, the strongest one I have. Kara is my greatest inspiration. She puts joy and laughter into my life.

There is a lovely old Victorian house in Melrose that sits on top of a hill; it has a magnificent view of Boston. Every time we pass by that place, I tell Tom and Kara that's my house. Tom announces, "You better start saving your pennies." Today Kara found a dirty brown and green penny on the ground that was all scratched up. She forfeited her discovery, and gave it to me. In her soft sweet voice, Kara nonchalantly said, "Mommy, you keep it. Save it for your house." Now tell me how a person can be down in the dumps with a special child like Kara!

I can allow myself to grieve about the cancer, and everything that comes with it including losing my baby. I know that in time, the blows will soften just like the frozen, winter earth in spring. I can let the tears flow. But I do not stay in that place for long. I did not make the decision to terminate my pregnancy to let it ruin my life. I did it to extend my life! I must reach for the power to go on living. I will not allow Jenna Rose's death to be in vein. I do not

Impossible Choices

want Tom or Kara to have more pain and sorrow. It is enough that they must deal with the cancer. I must show them that we are not defeated. I will be a happy wife and mother. They deserve this. And I deserve to be happy.

If I lose myself in my sorrow because I miss my baby so much, that would be a double tragedy. If I lose myself because I have cancer, that would be a real shame. If I stop living, if I enter into a deep depression, if I were to take drugs or alcohol to temporarily ease my pain, that would be disastrous! If I don't go on with my work, if I neglect myself and others, if I basically give up on life, that would be a surrender—two deaths. The real and actual death of my Jenna Rose, and the senseless, preposterous death of a living, breathing human being. I choose to embrace life and all that is beautiful around me. If I seek goodness instead of evil, I will heal my heavy heart. I choose to live. I choose to live happily ever after!!

May 26, 2000

Denise called today to tell me that she is pregnant with her third child. It was a difficult phone call for her to make, and she explained to me that she procrastinated for weeks because of my loss. She has two little boys and this baby is a girl. Of course she is thrilled. Denise is one of the kindest people I know. She has been my dear friend for seventeen years. She is six years my junior and I've always thought of her as the little sister I never had. I am glad for her and her husband. So many people don't know how to talk to me since the tragedy. Folks seem to be afraid to say the wrong thing. I have been in that predicament myself—worried that I would step all over my words. I guess it is always safe to speak from your heart. Silence hurts, and too much said is just that—too much said. Some middle ground is much appreciated. I am thankful

Denise was able to speak to me from her heart. I appreciate honesty.

May 29, 2000

I was up at Angel Hill and met another mother. We shared our sorrowful stories and cried together. When I got into the car, Kara asked me why I was crying. I answered her truthfully... that I missed our Jenna Rose. My sweet child said to me, "Mommy, don't be sad. You still have me." Yes, my Kara Elizabeth, I do have a most precious angel right here with me. I thought how very lucky I am; my sorrow evaporated instantly.

Our Kara loves Angel Hill where her baby sleeps. Kara plays with all the toys that rest on the gravesides of other babies. She carries stones, teddy bears, dolls, trucks, and anything else she can lift, carefully placing them on Jenna Rose's grave. When it is time to go home, she is very good about returning the belongings to their original sites. I have shed many tears at the site of these bittersweet memorials. I am careful to hold myself together in front of Kara. I am thankful that she does not understand the depth of what has happened to our family. We do not dwell on losing Jenna Rose because that would not be good for any of us, especially for Kara. My spirit lives in Kara. She is my angel here on earth. Jenna Rose is my angel in heaven.

May 31, 2000

I see how often I am the center of attention. Everything is focused on me and my illness. I wonder if folks realize how difficult it has been for Tom. He has been totally committed to me. My devoted husband continues to be a fortress of strength with his unconditional love and his unending support. He leaves the most

Impossible Choices

sentimental notes and greeting cards in places where they just pop out of nowhere. I have found them in my underwear drawer, kitchen cabinets, and countless other places. His love-notes and cards have me laughing and crying like a lunatic. I owe Tom so many back rubs that I'll never be able to repay him. Every night he gives me a terrific massage. His kneading and stroking always lead to foreplay, which ends in a night of passion. I have seen relationships crumble in times of crisis. I am most thankful that my marriage grows stronger and bolder with time. I love Tom more today than the day I married him, if that's even possible. We have reinforced our bond over and over again.

Our love is like a sapling which grows stronger each year. In the beginning, its young branches weather spring storms. Summer allows it to flourish and thrive. In the cold months it rests and sleeps and grows, gathering stamina for the year to come. Over time, the young larch expands round and firm, the sturdy boughs dividing and multiplying, extending tall into the air until it is the stalwart tamarack tree! This is how I see my marriage... my man... I am proud of him!

June 1, 2000

I sit alone this evening, here with my precious journal. It is late; the house is dark and quiet. My family dreams, but I am having another sleepless night. I have often considered how trivial some things really are. Things that before all this happened I would have worried about. I think of the people who get themselves upset over the tiniest matters, all because they are the biggest occurrences of their day. But I am learning much about myself and my inner strength. I still have a long journey ahead of me. I will continue on treatments of weekly Herceptin and chemotherapy until they stop

Barbara Dooling

working. I have completed three weeks of daily radiation to the femur, the original site of the largest and most painful tumor. Thankfully, I tolerate the chemotherapy treatments very well; I will have to receive them indefinitely. Each week I bring myself to the hospital to receive my magic potion. I wonder how I will do this for the rest of my life.

I had heard once that chemotherapy contained mustard gas from World War I. How terrifying is that? I remember back in 1997 the first time I was positioned in that seat waiting for the nurse to come and start the IV. Yah, there are rows of reclining blue chairs with little individual TV's attached to the wall behind each one. Everyone sits and waits and waits and waits and waits! You wait for the nurse and you bide time while the chemo drips, drips, drips. I remember how I cried fear my first time. Now, I'm an old pro. I can comfort other patients during their first experience. How often I have seen people crying! Some cry because they have cancer, others because they feel helpless. It is easy to think you have lost control of your life when you have to sit for hours while being infused with a drug that's supposed to save your life but that makes you extremely sick.

Although the procedure itself is time-consuming, sometimes there's an extra delay because of the hospital schedule. Too many people have cancer and the centers are overloaded! While you are waiting for an empty chair to receive your tonic, you can become very frustrated. When you have cancer, time becomes so precious to you. Folks who have the wicked "C" word dislike the feeling that they are wasting time. I have spent eight hour days at the mercy of chemotherapy and I have had to learn how to utilize that time. Mostly, I have spent the long treatment hours writing in Kara's journal. Other days I have gone visiting patients with my IV pole. I waltz

Impossible Choices

around looking for familiar faces and chat with my chemo buddies. It seems that when I help someone else feel better, that makes me better, too. These moments after sharing cancer stories, I do not feel alone with my troubles. Some exceptional people out there—like Mel, Betty, and Judy—have helped me to be optimistic. They are all my chemo comrades.

Once you've had a glimpse of death, you must rely on faith and hope to live. Sometimes it's better than any medicine. Despair will indeed make you lose power. We must bear in mind that we are all mortals, this includes the well and the sick. None of us can calculate how long we are destined to be here. We must spend our moments wisely. I have gained much inner strength knowing that I have touched the lives of fellow cancer patients. The threat of death has taught me plenty. I have learned that anyone living with cancer of any kind has courage. For any person who sits down in that chair and has chemotherapy infused into his or her body must be brave. To return each visit for more, takes backbone! To endure any serious illness with the side-effects takes stamina. There is the kind of dramatic courage when a firefighter rushes into a burning building to save a life. There is no denying he's a hero. But a cancer patient's courage is a quiet kind of day-to-day courage. To be a parent of a very sick child, watching helplessly as their little one suffers, is excruciating. These people, the patients and the parents, are extraordinary heroes.

June 18, 2000

I have just looked up the word "father" in the dictionary. We all know what the root of the word means and we all have a father. As I reflect on my life, I realize how very lucky I am to have such a great man for a father.

Barbara Dooling

My dad is not a wealthy man, but he is very rich in spirit. He loves his family with the greatest affection. The years brought difficult times for this ordinary man. There was the alcoholism which he found harder to lift from his life than those heavy weights when he was a champion. There was Mom's mental illness which dad suffered painfully as he watched his beautiful bride in so much anguish. Somehow the bond they shared, the commitment they had for one another, was the backbone of their marriage. Steadfast love and perseverance is what they raised their six children on.

Dad is a very sensitive man who can easily show his emotions. I have heard him say many times, that a man should not fear to cry. He has always, always yelled a lot. I think dad's way of crying is yelling. None of us children could ever stand his bellowing; Mom couldn't either. Perhaps he never saw himself as a big man and wanted to be heard. How often I should have told him, "We've listened to your valuable advice and taken to heart all you have taught us over the years." Somehow I don't think Dad will ever speak softly. I'm certain he will continue to shout loudly as long as he has a breath in him. It has always been his way.

My dad is a proud man and mostly proud of his children. His admiration has been clearly demonstrated over the years. He revels over our accomplishments, but mostly he just believed in the people we were. Recently Dad exhibited such pride when Russell received the very prestigious teacher's alumnus award. During Class Day 2000, at Dedham High, in an auditorium filled with students, parents, and teachers, Dad stood up when Russ was called to the stage to receive the award. This elderly man was so overwhelmed and proud of his son that he gave him a standing ovation. As I glanced around the auditorium, I knew Dad was the only person standing up. He was oblivious to this, and continued his

Impossible Choices

round of applause so firmly I thought he might fall over. As dad settled himself down in his chair, I couldn't help but cry. My tears fell for Dad. I was proud of my brother this day, but even more proud of my dad.

I love you, Daddy.

June 22, 2000

I am quite honored to be nominated facilitator of my breast cancer support group. Although I do my best administrating, this is not a job I do alone. We all manage the meetings, making it a peer run group. Our mission: to laugh and cry and learn things together. We even find humor in the despicable things related to our shared disease.

The group has taught me how to face cancer. I am inspired by each woman's fight against the same disease. There is a unique bond we all share. There are days when I need a good cry with someone else who has the cancer. It is not always so easy to ignore cancer. It badgers and torments day and night... dodging, shifting, and throwing punches. It never seems to be out of breath; it never seems to tire. It is hard to be in the ring with a prize fighter. We get shoved around a lot and knocked down. We have a right to our bad days, so long as we get back up again. So we learn the sly moves of a boxer and maybe we can even beat him!

I have formed a sisterhood with my group to escape from the side effects of cancer and its treatment. I have learned dozens of remedies for mouth sores, split nails, dry chaffed skin, and hot flashes, all of which are side effects from chemo. I have coped with neuropathy, the numbness and tingling in my fingers caused by chemo. I am cautious not to burn myself on the stove when I cannot feel heat. It is difficult to button my blouse and manipulate my fingers.

Barbara Dooling

The list goes on... Welts and head sores while your hair is falling out. I hadn't realized how useful our eyelashes are. Once I lost the protection of mine, my eyes became so dry that they stuck to my eyelids. I am constantly getting lint and dust and dirt in my eyes. It is painful. Who would have thought that the hair in your nostrils serves the wonderful purpose of keeping dust from making you sneeze. Moreover, those tiny hairs act like a washer for a leaky faucet, keeping body fluid from dripping out of your nose. When my nose is running, I have mere seconds to grab a tissue before the fluid pours out.

Let's see, what else? There's constipation and diarrhea all in the same week. Is that possible? Yes, it is. There is memory loss, better known as forgetful chemo brain. Ah, but why complain. We are still here! I mustn't forget how we all say the "f word" can ruin any good day—as in "f" for fatigue. Many of us get terrible fatigue with treatments. I'd rather keep taking my magic potion and cope with the side effects because the alternative is not good.

There are lots of pills for pain and side effects. Although when you take them, you wind up taking one more pill to counteract the effects of the other. Before you know it, you're taking thirty pills a day. The chemotherapy causes diarrhea and the pain medicines cause constipation. You wonder what message the brain will receive first. But, no matter what the side effects, I will grin and bear them as long as I can have my life in return.

Fear of cancer recurrence lives among most members, and those of us who have already metastasized fear death. Women of all ages worry about their families. It is most disturbing to think of our households getting along without us! The group has enlightened my vision. We rely on each other to get through. My lovely, caring earth angels have guided me with tremendous support and prayers

Impossible Choices

through the most difficult time in my life.

June 23, 2000

Walked the survivors lap with Ellen at the Relay for Life today! Had to. I'd promised myself and Ellen. Remember we were both going to be Prego's? She is seven months pregnant now and doing great! I am very happy for Ellen. This is her first baby. She deserves to have this baby. I'm not going to ask God again why I didn't deserve to have Jenna Rose? I can't think about it. I must push on! So… we walked and I cried the entire way around the track. I'm still here—still fighting!

June 29, 2000

My oncologist had great difficulty letting me know that she is pregnant. She struggled to make the announcement, probably not knowing what my reaction was going to be. We both cried and hugged each other. She asked if I wanted to be followed by another doctor. I am happy for her and I cannot hide from every pregnant woman. She will remain my doctor.

August 24, 2000

Jenna Rose was due this month! Oh God, I miss her. But I have been preoccupied with my health. See how God works? He puts me in the midst of turmoil but it must be for a reason! Ellen had her baby—a beautiful healthy boy! She is doing well with no signs of cancer recurrence. Go figure! Two women practically with the same diagnosis and prognosis. We both get pregnant, one does okay and the other is a huge disaster. Many other women besides Ellen have gone on to have healthy babies and normal pregnancies after being diagnosed with breast cancer. So what happened with me?

Barbara Dooling

I don't know! I just can't think about it… can't go there… nope… no can do! Got to move on. Got to fight this lousy cancer.

September 30, 2000

As if we haven't enough to contend with, Tom's company went on strike for six weeks. I am still in the five month waiting period with my state disability payments. My disability insurance from work has denied me the benefits because they are calling this breast cancer recurrence a preexisting condition. We virtually have no income. The stress has been piling up, load after load. Still, he finds room for humor. Tom says it's too bad I don't have any locks of hair to sell—we could use the money. Now that he's home all day, he wants to fool around and play doctor. He keeps stealing flowers out of the neighbors' yards. We have our own flowers and he picks those too. I think we both realize that all that matters is our health, with my recovery being the main focus. We try never to lose sight of this. Our days are spent laughing and loving each other.

We've had a few dinners of the old faithful—macaroni and cheese—but I served it on the good china! There's been French toast suppers and cereal by candlelight. Believe it or not, there is something memorable and inspirational about two people, completely in love, being able to share a supper of cereal by candlelight. We laughed through every bite.

Whatever else this life holds for us, however long I shall live, I shall not choose to spend it angry and grieving. I cherish our daughter Kara far too much to lose myself. I cherish Tom too, and I treasure our life together. Tom and I have remained totally committed through all of this, although our strength and love has been tested beyond limits. Love isn't real until it's been tested. How easy it is to be in love and how difficult to stay in love. It is only through

Impossible Choices

surviving the tempest, that we can claim our true love.

October 1, 2000

I'm sitting here thinking of the many, many physicians who have touched my life… and saved it! My doctors deserve a merit badge. They have my deepest gratitude; I feel so lucky to have found such quality care. They have demonstrated both expertise and human compassion. They guided me through an immense predicament, showing deep sincerity even to the point of shedding their own tears.

I am so appreciative of the nightingale nurses, tireless technicians, saintly secretaries and spirited staff members—even the vivacious volunteers! They make up a team equally important. Nurses seem to be the unsung heroes in medicine, working so closely with the physicians and patients. They are often extremely knowledgeable, compassionate, and experts at giving much needed hugs. My designated nurse Jyl is extraordinary in every sense of the word. I am grateful for her strong religious beliefs, providing me with great faith and hope. She is nonjudgmental and is committed to quality care, yielding unparalleled results. She delivers nothing short of the best! I thank any technician who has been courteous with me, taken the time to explain cumbersome tests, X-rays, and CT scans, and who have shown respect for my dignity! Secretaries and assisting staff members from file clerks to appointment coordinators, are not to be left out! I love how they are quick with a compliment on my new hair growth. I respect and appreciate all their efforts.

Let me not forget the dear, sweet volunteers. They are the sunshine people! These are folks who never stop smiling. These oldtimers (I pray they don't mind me calling them that) are young at heart. They are free-spirited people who are full of energy, skipping around the unit as though they are doing the polka. I envy their good health. Serving snacks, drinks, and lunch, is their specialty. However, these veterans of life have more to offer than sandwiches, juice, and tea!

October 7, 2000

Kara is almost four. Her daring play at the park has not changed much. I still worry for her. Daddy takes her hiking on a trail in the nearby woods. She has graduated to mountain climbing. I have scolded the two of them to stay off the rocks! Of course they did not heed my warnings, Kara wound up falling. Luckily she just got a few scrapes. My two rascals returned home with their tails between their legs. Kara was the brave one and spoke first, admitting her guilt fearlessly. I gave her a make-it-better kiss and hugged her tightly. Then I scolded again and again!

Like most young children, she is full of eternal energy. The chatter is nonstop, even in her sleep! She and I are often engaged in some imaginary play, pretending to be animals, doctors, veterinarians, kings, queens; you name it. Funny, I am always the poor sick patient, the hurt dog, or the queen's servant. You guessed it; when we play Cinderella, I'm either the wicked stepmother or the mean, nasty stepsister! She plays all the leading characters and there is no negotiating the roles. She is more merciful to her playmates. Her friends can be whomever they choose, but Mom is assigned the part that Kara picks. She is just too funny!

October 12, 2000

Kara is enrolled in preschool two days a week. Separation has been very difficult for both of us. I am assured by her teachers that

Impossible Choices

she has a "great day" once I leave. But then at bedtime, she continues to inform me that she dislikes going to school. Drop off has always been quite the scene with lots of crocodile tears and leg clutching. I leave the school crying, too. Who wouldn't with a little one screaming out, "Mommy, Mommy don't leave me!" Each day I remind her about all of her new friends in Ms. Robin and Ms. Mary's class, and the crafts, activities and singing. I tell her it isn't necessarily school that she dislikes, it's the fact that Mommy has to leave. No, she insists that she doesn't like a thing about school!

Nightmares have started, and in the morning she cries out from her bed, "Mommy, is this a school day?" I gingerly answer, "Yes, Lovey. Today you get to play with all your friends." Kara returns with a plea, "I want to change the day!" Daddy and I hold back our laughter, and I sympathetically answer, "I know, Bear Cub, Mommy would like to change the day too sometimes, but we can't." I put little surprises inside her lunch box. Sometimes I put a cute card, a note from me or her daddy, a picture of our family, or some little treat. We have a new routine at the school where she watches me from the window and waves good-bye as I climb into the car. I taught her the I-love-you hand signal in sign language. She has mastered it beautifully. How adorable she looks while she struggles with her tiny fingers, trying to fold them just so. She studies her hand intently, looking down until she gets it right… then she catches my gaze out the window. I return the sign, get into my car, and cry.

Another thing we do is to read a wonderful book called *The Kissing Hand*. This is a story about a baby raccoon who must go to school and he, too, misses his mommy. The mommy raccoon kisses her baby's paw and tells him to place it to his cheek whenever he is sad and missing her. So in the morning, I smother Kara's little hand with bunches of kisses for the day. She in turn kisses my

Barbara Dooling

hand, leaving me with hers throughout my day. These routines work quite well.

November 1, 2000

Ever since our lives have been turned upside down by cancer, I have tried to keep Kara's routines consistent. Despite everything, I want Kara to have stability in her life. She was just a baby when I was first diagnosed with breast cancer. It wasn't necessary to explain anything about the illness to her at that time. I had hoped that it would just be one of those things from the "past" that I would one day tell her about when she was older. Now that the cancer is back and here to stay, there is a need to explain specifics as they come along. She is older and full of questions about the changes it has brought. Although she is inquiring more about the cancer, I am glad she is still too young to understand the magnitude and potential threat of my illness. Nevertheless, I must introduce her to cancer.

We talk about it, but I make the conversations brief. She is too little to bombard with information which is meaningless to her. We try to maintain her routines, and we keep her up-to-date with the doctor updates and treatments. Her daddy and I always answer her questions honestly. The most difficult concept for Kara is that Mommy's illness isn't going away. She sees me continue to take medicine and go to the doctors frequently. She knows that Mommy goes to treatment every week and I am gone all day.

Common words used in our house are *radiation*, *chemotherapy*, *doctor*, and *nurse*. Kara knows that although Mommy's medicine is supposed to help her, it sometimes makes her tired and sick. The medicine also makes her hair fall out. When I explained to her that I was going to shave my remaining hair, she feared she would not

Impossible Choices

recognize me. "Mommy, don't take all your hair off because I won't know who you are." That's when we had our "Mommy to Kara" talk. I told her that she would know my face... that I'm still her mommy with or without hair... that I would love her always, and she will see that love in my eyes. I would love her with my smile, and she would hear my affectionate words. I would love her with my arms and they would embrace her with care. I would love her with all my heart, and its rhythm would beat her name. Then I let her play with my wigs and hats. We got silly and laughed. She has learned not to pull Mommy's wig off in the stores! That's right... we take the wig off once we get home, not in the stores! Ha, ha. Yep, Kara tried to take my wig off in the supermarket. She's one smart girl because she knows it comes off.

Kara has learned what a portacath is, and she has seen how it works. Mommy has taken her to treatments where she watched the nurses insert a special needle with long tubing into my port. She knows this is how I get the chemotherapy. She calls it "chemo" just like everyone else. She has learned to be careful not to bang or press down on my port. She has her own doctor kit, and practices advanced medicine on her dollies and stuffed animals. Most children play with the pretend stethoscope and thermometer. They know what these things are. Kara administers chemo to her babies. Kara performs surgery and minor procedures on her dolls! My little one is such a sponge.

This is one area in which I wish she wasn't so educated. But we must keep her involved in my care. I don't want her to be afraid of the unknown. When I came home from the hospital with staples in my leg, she was terrified to sit next to me. It is no wonder because the staples are scary looking. It was the same with the portacath. She was quite worried about the lump it created on Mommy's chest. I let her know that it was okay for her to ask questions and tell me her fears. I thought about my answers and explanations before I talked with her. I assured her these places on Mommy's body did not hurt. I never forced unwanted discussions or physical contact, and she eventually touched the staples and the port on her own. She knows that the staples are temporary, and the port is permanent.

I have often wondered if I tell her too much. After all, she is only four years old. But children are naturally curious. These are everyday situations in our home. I feel that her questions are her way of letting us know that she is ready to hear the answer. Though it is often difficult to explain such complicated and serious matters, she is not aware that they are complicated and serious. She has no idea that other children do not know what a port is. We must learn to trust our judgment. Tom and I must teach her how to cope with my illness. Although it's instinctual to want to shelter Kara, and keep her away from the hurt, we need to guide and direct her. If we raise our daughter totally in the dark, we risk her tripping and getting hurt anyway. Teaching Kara how to overcome problems as they come up will hopefully keep her path clear of stumbling blocks.

December 9, 2000

We went to the grave today to bring a small Christmas tree and trinkets to decorate the headstone. Kara is too young to feel the deep sorrow Tom and I feel after losing the baby. Kara is so curious as to what heaven is all about. We hardly bring her to the cemetery anymore—we never really brought her much in the first place. If she asks, we take her. Kara tells me that she doesn't like heaven. She claims that it is not a good place. Wow, do I have some explaining to do. She keeps asking me for a sister or brother. It breaks my

Impossible Choices

heart.

Kara has told perfect strangers that Mommy had a baby in her belly, and it died. She has asked Mommy and Daddy what happened to our baby and why we can't have another one. And I think that warrants an answer. I explained to her that my body was too sick to carry the baby. Kara told me that when she gets a baby in her belly, it's not going to die. That's right, Kara, I sure hope so!

December 10, 2000

I explained to my sweet child that heaven is certainly a wonderful place. I agreed with her that she might feel that she has good reason to dislike heaven because heaven is keeping her from holding her baby sister Jenna Rose, but that perhaps we can hold Jenna Rose in other ways. Like whenever we hold and pet a soft fluffy baby bunny or kitten, we are holding Jenna Rose. That Jenna Rose's body might not be here, but that her spirit is very close-by protecting us. I tried to explain that heaven is a divine paradise that keeps Jenna Rose very safe and comforted, a place high above in the heart of God, where she can watch over us and share our lives in a different kind of way.

Maybe one day Kara will understand this better than she does now. I will keep trying to explain it all whenever the opportunity presents itself. See? I still have lots to teach her and I need to be here on earth to do that! She asked me if I am going to die and be in heaven with our baby. She implored that she wanted to go to heaven too and asked, "Mommy, will there be room in heaven for me?" Mommy explained that heaven is as big as the universe. I told her to just look at the huge blue sky. And I said that someday we will all go to heaven. But for right now, Kara and Mommy and Daddy are going to live together here on earth for as long as we can. I am constantly amazed at her questions.

December 23, 2000
    The cancer is relentless; it knows no boundaries! It has progressed in my bones and the pain leaves me weak. God, I sure hope this chemo is still working. On some recent X-ray films, the right femur appears to be collapsing. This causes the hip to hurt as well. My walking is atrocious and I limp because one leg is shorter than the other. I struggle with housework and it is impossible to lift Kara. This is beginning to be a bummer all over again. It is wretched keeping ahead of the cancer. But we have special people who love us and are just as persistent as my disease! I have never asked myself, "What did I ever do to deserve the cancer?" Rather I have asked, "What did I ever do to deserve such wonderful family and friends?" I am surrounded by an abundance of family kindness and golden friendships. I have harvested more than I have sowed.

    Bruce, Mary, and Aunt Phyilis and Uncle Lawrence have all donated money to start a trust fund for Kara. Julie comes to chemo each week to sit with me while it drips, drips, drips. Sheila—good ol' Sheila, my lifelong friend—treated us to an all-expense-paid vacation to Disney World, Florida! I can't believe we'll finally get to take Kara to my favorite place! It's going to be such a special trip for us!

    An ophthalmologist Elliot, who shared the same suite with my boss, presented me with a splendid gift. He and his daughter and partner Macie awarded me a brand new computer and printer. And Elliot's wife Betty suggested that I write a book on the computer! That's a thought. I remember receiving a father-like hug from Elliot when I was pregnant and learned that the cancer had metastasized. I cried in his arms when I told him the news, and I believe he was

Impossible Choices

crying, too. And now I am crying all over again. Thanks you guys, from the bottom of my heart. I will write that book, Betty, absolutely. How can I ever thank you enough for such a gift? I know, I will show my appreciation by making sure I write that book!

People have been so good to me—to us. The only way I know how to repay such giving is with my open heart. I am truly blessed.

December 27, 2000

Disney world was amazing. Thank you, Sheila, you are the greatest! What a delight to see the wonder in Kara's face as she met all of her favorite characters. She was so full of excitement! It certainly brought out the inner child in us, too! It was truly magical. How fortunate to have this time together. I cried each of the four days we spent at Disney. I was so moved—torn between happiness and sadness. Mostly, I was happy to be with my family… my very own family at Disney World. Wahoo! This is yet another blessing. So many cherished gifts to balance all the pain. In fact, every morning I wake up is a bright and glorious gift—the gift of a new day!

January 22, 2001

The weirdest thing happened today. I saw a puffy cloud that looked just like a baby. At first I thought I was going crazy. Usually I see elephants and other types of animals in the clouds. Never have I seen the shape of a baby up there in all my life. A shiver ran through my entire body. I called Tom to come outside quickly for his opinion. I questioned, "Is it me or do you see a baby in that cloud, too?" For sure, it is! Tom said it looked like a cherub. We stood together in silence, staring up at the sky in wonderment. I am certain that we shared the very same thought: Jenna Rose was

Barbara Dooling

saying hello from heaven.

February 23, 2001

Today we took a ride to good old White Horse Beach. Brrrrrr! No matter how cold it is, we find an opportunity to bundle up and head for the ocean to play. During the winter months, the water looks charcoal black with frosted white caps. There are only a few lonely seagulls soaring through the sky. They balance in the air, hovering, ready to scavenge their food. I hear them crying news to each other. The wind is constantly blowing. It never ceases to whip across the beach depositing sand like snow drifts. Atlantic blasts nip at any exposed skin. Your nostrils freeze and eyes tear from the frigid bitterness. Not many folks dare to battle these harsh elements. One must really love the sea! Today, as I gazed upon the dark water, I traveled deep into my thoughts, focusing on my cancer fears and my cancer pain.

My daydream is fresh in my mind: rocks and gravel huddled at the shoreline, rolling up onto the beach. I stand as close to the water's edge as the waves allow without getting soaked. I find myself a stick and write the word C A N C E R in the firm sand. I wait and watch as the waves wash away this nasty word. Staring out on the horizon where the ocean meets the sky, I drift with those white caps into conscious sedation. Screeches and laughter from Kara and Tom become muffled; I lose track of where they are.

Lost in my daydream, I imagine myself a captain on a huge ship with puffing, canvas sails. I picture myself battling a fierce ocean storm. There is much beauty in the raging sea, even though I fear the storm. My mind drifts like the water. I visualize an ebony sky that lights up with each jagged strike of lightning. The claps of thunder are deafening. My vessel is colliding with the wild, breaking

Impossible Choices

waves. What do I do? How do I survive this? Choices… choices… I have to make choices! I must figure a way to survive. Will I make the right decisions? Will I do the correct things that will lead me to safety? Or will I perish?

In my dream, I wonder how long the storm will last. When I am exhausted from fighting the turbulent waters and wild winds, when the darkness seems like an eternity, and I fear I can bear no more, suddenly the brilliant sun rises beyond the depths of the now calm tide. Before me sprawls the glistening ocean, and the once powerful waves are nearly still. Swells are a mere ripple. I can only hear them softly flowing. I look along the horizon. The blackened sky has turned crimson pink and lilac purple. I am even blessed to see part of a rainbow; the other arch is hidden beneath the few remaining clouds. There are no more forceful chilling gusts driving against my back. There is only a warm breeze, which feels, gentle and feathery on my face. I am grateful for the splendid view before me. There is a profound silence within me.

I smile. I am at peace. I am alive. In some strange way, I have been inspired by this powerful struggle. Endurance has brought courage I never knew existed within myself. I will respect all that has happened, even the assault, because it has changed my life. My wild imagination is interrupted by Kara's bellows. She is calling, "Mommy! Mommy! Mommy, come play with us!" I must get back to shore and dock this vessel. I am back to reality. I did love the voyage though. I will play an active roll in my treatment while I concentrate and focus on recovery. I must choose the way I wish to live my life. When things discourage me, I will pretend that I am sailing a ship across the wild blue ocean. I will perceive the challenge differently… positively… as an adventure that is to be mastered. Nothing will break my spirit; I shall not be defeated. I will be victorious no matter what the outcome. The battlefield is in my mind, not the body, and I am the master of my mind.

Ahoy! Good luck to me! Cast away care, Mate! I'll secure the hatch, stand guard, and hold a steady course! I am seaworthy, and I will reach that port! I will anchor and rest myself in the shelter of the harbor!

My daughter continues to interrupt with her shouting. She summons me. I smile and salute the sea. "I'll be right there, Sweetie!"

February 28, 2001
Oops, forgot to mention... Started my book a few months ago. I'm going to do it "my" way—just polish up my journal and take excerpts and string them together into a novel. *Voila!*

March 1, 2001
Since I met Father Mike one year ago, I welcome our weekly meetings. I am thankful that the Mass General has a priest like him. I have never had the opportunity to share conversation with a priest week after week. I have been so privileged to do so with my wonderful new friend Father Mike. When I attend church in my own congregation, I am usually greeted by the clergy at the end of the mass with a handshake. There is always a full procession of people scuffling through towards the exit. It is hard to exchange more than a few casual words. I have never engaged in parish council with the exception of this past spring when I revealed my pregnancy and cancer dilemma to our priests. At that time, I feared being banned from the catholic church because of my situation.

I am not a habitual Sunday observer, but I consider myself someone who practices her faith. I believe in eternal life because I

Impossible Choices

believe in God. I rely on my faith almost daily. Even before I got cancer, I always talked to God. When I informed the priests at my own parish that we were facing the decision to terminate my pregnancy, I was relieved that they did not judge me. Perhaps they felt that this judgment was best left up to God. They were, in fact, quite sympathetic to the problem. I received their prayers and blessings. We did not meet again. Now each week when Father Mike is here, I am overcome with calm. His conversation is genuine and comforting. His manner is mild and pleasant. I have learned so much from him over these months. I am thankful for the communion he brings to the chemo unit. The Eucharist heals me spiritually.

I have not been able to bring myself back to church since I terminated the pregnancy nearly one year ago. I cannot bear to look at the mahogany font where our baby would have been baptized. I recollect how this phobia started. It was shortly before Easter last year, and our parish had just been renovated. A new mahogany font was placed at the entrance of the church aisle. Palm Sunday was the first mass held in the upstairs since the completion of a year long restoration. I attended mass with Tom and Kara. We were still agonizing over the predicament. As I walked into the church that Palm Sunday, my eyes were fixed on the brand new, intricately designed wooden font. I was mesmerized by its beauty. I was five months pregnant with Jenna Rose. I wept through the entire Palm Sunday mass. Our baby was never to be baptized in that font!

Because I would have to walk past the font to enter the church, I have not been able to attend masses since that day. Therefore, I have been unable to celebrate with the Holy Eucharist. Father Mike's weekly visits at the Mass General have allowed me this sanctity, and with it my faith has been restored. I have absorbed his humanity and schooling on theology. He has been like an apostle, preaching the gospel, and I have been his disciple. I think of him with deepest appreciation. I don't know how I would get along without him.

April 22, 2001
Happy Birthday to me! Wow! I'm forty and loving it! That's because I'm still here on this earth with my beautiful family and caring friends. Tom has outdone himself once again. Jeez, with so much going on with my cancer care, he still found time to plan a surprise fortieth birthday party! His love is forever. I have the tallest giant for a husband and the richest life a woman could ever dream of! Today Tom entertained me along with one hundred and thirty people at a local hall here in Melrose. It was like a small wedding! I just kept crying all day as I hugged family, friends, doctors, and nurses—all my greatest fans! My life is incredibly rich indeed! This was the day of all days with my true love Tom was all over it! And my sweet child Kara Elizabeth running and dancing wildly all over the dance floor. All my favorite people who I love so very much were there to wish me the happiest birthday!

May 1, 2001
I am scheduled to have my femur bone replaced since it is collapsing. The orthopedic oncologist will remove the screws that hold my leg together and put a titanium rod through the femur. More surgery! Well, it has to be done since I can barely function with this darn pain. Forget the pain pills they give me... half of them don't work, and they all make me so sick. I cannot take narcotics because I vomit profusely. I don't know what is worse, the nausea or the pain. It is a vicious circle... when I can't bare the pain

Impossible Choices

anymore, I resort to the drugs. Then I get so sick to my stomach that I'm laid up in bed for hours. The anti-nausea drugs don't seem to help. I guess the surgery is a must!

May 9, 2001

The book is coming along. I've transferred many journal entries into my new computer. I can't help wondering if these passages will really become a novel fit for publishing. I'm committed to see it through. I have withstood the crushing blows of disaster and disappointment. My writing is just one of the ways I have coped. Here on these pages I can diffuse pain, anger, and sadness without losing hope. If anything comes of this writing, I shall be ecstatic. My greatest dream is that one day Kara will read a book that her mother wrote especially for her. She will see first hand that we do not have to be defeated by life's betrayals. And we cannot close ourselves off for fear of further pain.

May 13, 2001

Another Mother's Day—the second since losing Jenna Rose. Today I visited her grave by myself. A pesky little squirrel has been digging up the soil, antagonizing the crocus bulbs that Tom planted last fall. There are plenty of acorns scattered on the ground, yet the little rascal prefers to disturb our flower bed. She greeted me today, upon my arrival. I shooed her away. She hopped boldly on top of Jenna's headstone and stared at me with black beady eyes. Neither one of us dared to move. Then I decided to talk to that gray ball of fur. She actually chirped a reply. That squirrel sat perched the whole twenty minutes I was there. Hello, my little Jenna Rose… yes, there's no doubt in my mind you would have been keeping me on my toes, getting into all kinds of mischief. I love you my little queen

Barbara Dooling

of mischief.

May 23, 2001

Great! Another complication! Just great! The surgery has been postponed because I have been suddenly diagnosed with a heart condition called cardiac myopathy, which is a weakening of the heart muscles! What next? During a test called a Gated Heart Scan, a scan that shows heart function by measuring what is called the ejection fraction, they found that my heart muscles are not pumping the blood properly. It is routinely given to people who are taking the antibody Herceptin because the drug has a possible side effect of damaging the heart muscles. Along with chemotherapy I have been taking Herceptin antibody every week since April 2000.

Once we learned of the cardiac myopathy, I was immediately sent to a cardiologist who now has me on three heart medicines and recommended I stop the Herceptin. He has also advised me not to have any surgery, namely the leg surgery, for three months unless it is an emergency. After an echocardiogram and a day spent in the hospital for two procedures, it has now been confirmed that chemotherapy has damaged my heart. The cardiologist performed a catheterization through the main artery in my groin and a heart biopsy through the Corotid artery in my neck. The two procedures were unpleasant, but I did go home at the end of the day!

The biopsy actually shows deposits on the heart muscle from the previous Chemotherapy I took back in 1997. Adriamycin. Apparently there are certain cells left on the heart in a pattern that are characteristic for Adriamycin. There is no evidence of the Herceptin, on my heart. However this drug can also cause damage. I've been told that Herceptin is still too new of a drug and not enough is known about it. Although other chemotherapy drugs can

Impossible Choices

cause cardiac myopathy, namely Adriamycin, the Herceptin very well could have instigated this problem.

It is permanent! Despite the fact that I will have this condition for the rest of my life, it can be controlled with heart medication. I should regain most of the heart function back with time. The frightening part for me is coming off the Herceptin. That is my drug! This also cuts my chemotherapy list since many of the chemo drugs can affect the heart. As Gilda Radner said, "It's always something."

I said to Tom, in a bit of a sarcastic tone, "Boy, you sure picked yourself a winner for a wife!" Why does something always trip me up every time I begin to run? How come the hurdle gets knocked down as I'm leaping over it? My sweet Tom replied, "I did pick me a winner. I got first prize! I got the gold medal!" He's incredible! He's one big reason I keep fighting, with a coach like him, who wouldn't? So I get up, I dust myself off and I keep running.

June 30, 2001

I've had the most wonderful opportunity to visit with a group of Carmelite nuns in New York City. It all came about because I needed a place to stay while I went to Memorial Sloan Kettering Hospital for a second opinion. My cousin Debbie knows the nuns, and asked that she and I lodge at the convent during our brief two days in Manhattan. I am in search of any clinical trials for metastatic breast cancer that may seem hopeful. Although my appointment at Sloan proved to be informative, it was also disappointing because I do not fit the criteria for any of their trials. I was however, reassured that I am getting excellent medical care in Boston. Staying with the Carmelite sisters was the most enlightening part of the trip. Each one of them lifted me in prayer and gave me hope. They have amazing zeal! I was spiritually moved by their astounding faith. I was so grateful to them, and to Debbie for taking such good care of me. Debbie had to push me around in a wheel chair on the streets of New York in ninety-eight degree weather because I'm in too much pain to walk even the slightest distance. She pampered me with flowers and catered to my every need. Despite this restful mini-vacation, which seemed more like a retreat, I was missing my Tom and Kara.

July 6, 2001

The wait is on for my surgery! For the entire month of June through the Fourth of July celebrations, the pain in my leg has grown progressively worse. I am mentally and physically drained from the pain. I can't bear the weight of walking. How am I ever going to wait through these three months until my heart improves? What choice do I have?—NONE. The end of June was the Relay for Life! This was my second year! Yep, I hobbled around that track with Ellen! She brought her little boy to the relay. He'll be a year old next month; my Jenna Rose would have been that old too. And guess what? Ellen is pregnant again with twins! How incredible is that? It's been a few weeks since I walked the victory lap and I've been in so much agony; I am nauseous. I think my hip must be broken.

July 12, 2001

Oh my God, it is broken! The X-ray today revealed that the head of the femur is gonzo—collapsed and my hip has indeed fractured! Oops, guess that walk around the track did me in! Just another setback. I desperately need the leg surgery. It's now an emergency! The cardiologist has given his approval for the estimated six hour total hip and femur replacement, providing I have no anesthesia. I will undergo these procedures with an epidural. Oh wonderful! More

Impossible Choices

procedures without anesthesia.

July 16, 2001

I should be used to this by now. I was given ear plugs and head phones! I was awake! The epidural was for the pain and they gave me some valium intravenously which worked well to keep me calm. I swear I could heard the saw cutting my femur and hip! I drifted in and out of sleep. What an ordeal!

July 30, 2001

The surgery was a wonderful success and I am walking and driving with no pain! Yep, after a whole year, I am pain free! Recovery has been speedy and the doctors are all quite pleased. No one is as psyched as me! Yahoo! New body parts and I feel great!

August 1, 2001

I've been at the computer night and day fitting together the pieces of my life! The book is shaping up. I've started looking for publishers. This is a whole new world for me—the industry and the procedure of submitting a manuscript. It's like learning a new language. We shall see how far I get. Fortunately, I do have one connection... not that connections work in the publishing world, especially for new authors. But I will try. That's one positive thing about cancer... you're not afraid to reach. You have nothing to lose.

August 10, 2001

A beautiful yellow butterfly landed on Kara's shoulder today! Kara instantly froze to keep from frightening the dainty cheerful creature away. How bright and delicate her wings! Kara kept whispering, "Look, Mommy, the flutterby is dancing on my shoulder!" I winked at the butterfly. Hi Jenna Rose, how nice of you to remind Kara that you are her faithful companion. Thanks for enjoying this fine day with us.

August 13, 2001

Lost a member of the support group today—Karen. The cancer went to her liver, now she's dead. God, don't let it go to my liver and kill me! I went to see her a few days ago. Not sure how I was able to put myself through that. It was like sitting with Annmarie when she was dying. But, I had to say good-bye. I know that there will be an empty feeling in all of us in the group for a long time. Karen was a beautiful person who we all loved. She had sparkling eyes and a hearty laugh. She was kind and caring, and she loved her family very much. We'll miss her.

September 9, 2001

I am nearing the completion of my book and have found a lovely woman Diane Reagan to edit my grammar. I am grateful to her for tackling the huge task of getting my manuscript ready for a publisher! I literally called her into my life one day, and she graciously accepted. She did not know this stranger who asked her to help correct punctuation, verb tense, and sentence structure in a book about a cancer journey. However, she willingly ventured to my home to learn about me, my family, and my book.

It was charitable of her to do the job without getting paid for her precious time. I am indebted to her. How generous to say that this was her contribution to a good cause. As she knew from reading my manuscript, I had had an outpour of help from friends and relatives. But she is someone who did not even know me. She is one of those caring people who make the world a better place.

Impossible Choices

As she and I worked together, I felt like I was back in school again. I was frustrated when she suggested I "change the order of paragraphs, shorten a run-on sentence, or find a better word." Not to mention, the paragraphs that she said needed "clarification." Evidentially it was clear to me but not my reader. I know the perfect stocking stuffer for her this year: a red marker.

Despite my flaws, she was equally as generous with her compliments. It was uplifting to read her approving remarks. Her praise helped me to have confidence. My book is compiled of many feelings, both happy and sad. It was beneficial to hear her opinion about the way it was written. I value her judgment and trust her advice. Now that the project is nearly complete, I know that we will remain good friends. It would be nice to get together for a social visit and not have to talk about English grammar. I promised her that I would keep my comas, semicolons, and colons straight. My verbs and tenses will need improvement, but I shall be cautious of those as well.

She is one fine person with a big heart. I shall not forget all that she has done for me. Her time and efforts are much appreciated. I hope that it's true that what you give out, you get back tenfold. She deserves a millionfold.

September 19, 2001

Another friend perished from this God forsaken breast cancer! My good friend Linda, she was only forty-four and she leaves behind a little four year old. My heart breaks for that little boy! My heart breaks for Kara. Please God, please let me live. I spent an awful lot of time with Linda before she died. I called her just about every day. We would reminisce about going on picnics with the children. She and I had a lot of lunches at the parks this past spring when she was

Barbara Dooling

doing well with the cancer. Then, suddenly, without warning, the cancer spread to her brain. No, please don't let it go to my brain. Poor Linda was so fragile—she just couldn't fight anymore. She became so ill, and within a few weeks, she was dying. I went to her bedside and wept with her. I held her hand while she told me she did not want to leave her son. Her ivory skin was transparent—like Annmarie's. Her lips cracked and bleeding—like Annmarie's. She labored for every breath. Her chest, rising and falling with clumsy hard respiration, puffing and panting with each short breath. Yep, it was all the same watching her die, too!

Tom was angry. He didn't want me going over to Linda's house. He didn't want me to see her that way. They radiated her brain... What? Why? To give her a few more weeks? That nearly killed her anyway. She was like a vegetable; she was so tired and weak. Her hair... gone again. It came out in clumps. Linda. She was so pretty. She had engaging eyes and a happy, happy smile. She had jet black hair... well, okay... it was a little gray, too. She was tall and slender. God, when the weight came off her she looked like a skeleton. Where am I going with all of this? I haven't a clue. Linda's husband and her mother... so distraught! Her boy... so confused! Tom was probably right, it did me no good to be there. But I had to be there for my friend. Good-bye, Linda. I shall miss you.

September 28, 2001

I have started a new chemotherapy drug Xeloda, which I seem to be tolerating well. The disease has spread to more areas in my bones. I received this news just last week. I have progression of the disease in some places and new lesions (cancer spots) in other areas. This information is unsettling to say the least, but the good news is that my liver is clean and my lungs are stable. I have had a

Impossible Choices

tiny spot in my right lung since last year which has remained unchanged. Basically, I'm on a plateau. I am treading water—at least staying afloat. I never could swim. I've had lessons many times, but I'm actually a very poor swimmer. I am quite afraid of the water. So I'm a drifter. But that's okay because I'll take that rather than sinking!

The bony metastasis, as they call it, is at times painful. I am praying that the new chemotherapy works. I had been on the former drug Taxol, since April 2000 with the Herceptin antibody. I received that regimen each week during a five hour infusion. The Xeloda is a pill that I take at home! Yippee! I am disappointed to be forced to take another new drug, but it does have its advantages. I will also have hair again! Evidentially, this drug does not make your hair fall out!

The disadvantage to changing drugs is of course, new side effects. But the main problem is that failing a treatment means loss of longevity with that drug. There are only so many treatments for breast cancer and you want to get the most out of each one. So I move onto another therapy and hope for the best. It is all I can do! That, and pray! I will continue my fight against the enemy. Cancer is a fierce opponent. Sometimes I am tired. But I must keep going!

Besides the goings on with cancer, chemotherapy, and surgery we did have a great summer. The weather was simply gorgeous. We vacationed twice in Maine and spent much of that time at the beach. Kara had a grand time splashing in the cold water, chasing and running from waves, building and smashing sand castles, collecting and tossing rocks and seashells, and running along the beach. I had a grander time watching her. This was how she entertained herself and us in between kicking sand on the blanket or reaching into the cooler with sand-caked hands. Beach etiquette must be something you acquire when you're older?

September 30, 2001

Hey, I peeked in the mirror and I look pretty good if I do say so myself! I have lost eighteen pounds in the past few months, but I've gained eight back. Life with Tom and Kara continues to be a great joy. I am quite proud of my little family. As the steamy hot summer days give way to cool autumn breezes, I am thankful to be alive. Sharing these beautiful days with my family, is such an inspiration. I know that my family and friends all continue to keep us in their thoughts and prayers.

October 2, 2001

I take a moment to recognize my former boss Andy. Not only was he such a good boss, but he has been my friend. I appreciate that he still keeps in touch with me after I left on disability in March of 2000.

How generous... he has added to the trust fund for our Kara Elizabeth! The money was more than charitable. Tom and I are both astonished, and we are most grateful to him. Now that I am on disability, surviving cancer has become my full time job. It does not pay very well, but the benefits are excellent. I get to live if I do my job well.

During the seven years that I was his medical office manager, our work relationship had its ups and downs. But mainly, we had very few disagreements. We honestly respected each other, and we functioned rather well together. We made a strong team.

In 1997 when I was first diagnosed with breast cancer, I returned to work just two weeks after my surgery. I continued working through my chemotherapy and daily radiation treatments.

Impossible Choices

Though he was more than willing to give me time off, I know that he appreciated my efforts to keep the continuity in his practice. He always showed concern for me. I have learned that many employers are not as understanding when their employee has a serious illness. This can be a real problem for people with cancer. I had always loved my job. I enjoyed the medical profession and working with people. And I really liked working with Andy. I miss him.

Not only is Andy a fine eye surgeon and ophthalmologist, but he is caring and compassionate to all of his patients. I became spoiled by the way he treated his patients, and I now I expect this same considerate attention from my own doctors. It was not out of the ordinary for Andy to send sympathy cards to the family of a patient who had passed away. It was not unusual for him to check in on his patients after hours or over a weekend. I remember he drove to one of his patient's homes in a snowstorm and drove her to the Mass Eye and Ear Infirmary so she could have her cataract surgery. He sends flowers to his patients after their surgery!

Actually, not flowers—big potted plants! He was equally giving to his employees. Dinner and the theater were not unusual perks in his practice. Coffee, muffins, and lunch were a sporadic treat. And it was not an uncommon gesture for him to battle a windy and torrential rainstorm to deliver a barely-used bicycle to our home before Christmas Day. His younger daughter's old bike was still in excellent condition, and he shined it up, and gave it to Kara. These are the kind gestures that single him out! Again, I reflect on such beautiful people in my life.

October 5, 2001

Today I called a publisher! I gave the contact name like my contact told me to, and all the information about this growing book of mine. I just don't know. The publisher was in London and sounded very busy. She explained that the only reason why she had returned my call was because my contact was very dear to her. She lamented that a book about cancer was not the most marketable subject matter, and that the company was overloaded with projects. She did listen to me explain about my personal struggles with cancer and I could tell that she was empathetic about my situation... but... but she also said that lots of people call with pleas to publish their books about their personal struggles. She would have to think about it, but that it was not likely to be a match for their list. What a bummer. This is going to be a miserable journey.

How incredible! The publisher called back and explained that a rainbow had been splashed across the sky out her window after hanging up the phone with me. She went on to say that at first she lowered the blinds on the rainbow because she was overwhelmed with projects and didn't want her decision to be influenced by the rainbow... but that the rainbow had continued to nag at her after it had evaporated. She told me to send the manuscript and she would take a look.

November 5, 2001

Two new angels flew into my life. Ironically they both have the same name—Mel. I met them on different occasions at the hospital. Mel from Maine has had bone cancer for nine years; I met her in the waiting room of my orthopedic oncologist. She is the sweetest, most vibrant young woman! She talks a mile a minute, and she lights up the room with her huge cheerful smile. I think we are going to be good friends. We will keep in touch by letters and phone, and when Tom and I go to the cottage in Maine, we can visit

Impossible Choices

her and her family.

The other Mel is just as nice and full of spice! I met her during chemo! She had just completed treatment for breast cancer—luckily she has not metastasized. Mel number two is a hoot! She cracks me up. But all jokes aside, she has taken me under her wing, and adopted me as a special friend. I've only known her a short time and the woman keeps showering me with gifts. She shows up unannounced on my chemo days and brings fresh baked cookies and breads. To top it off, she has given me a card spiked with two, one hundred dollar bills! She must be crazy! She wants me to have a night out on the town with Tom—on her! Good Lord! We can have dinner, drinks, dancing and dreams at a hotel for that money! Who is this angel that God has sent me? She is amazing! Even though we've just met, I feel as though we've been friends for years! What a Sweetie!

December 1, 2001

This gallant man I married is courageous and noble! How often he has cleared my tears with his words and his tenderness. I believe him whole heartedly when he tells me that beauty is truly in the eye of the beholder. When we first met, and he rented the movie, *Beauty and The Beast*, it was a foreshadowing of our own life. Here we are, ten years since the day we met. I have lost my hair for the third time since my diagnosis. My body reveals two scars where tumors were taken out. The chemotherapy treatments have stolen the flush coloring right out of my face. A jaundice shade replaces my pink cheeks. My eyelashes and eyebrows are gone, completely bare. My body is weary and I no longer stand straight. Not only has the chemotherapy deprived me of energy, but the cancer attacks my body, withering my bones like those of an aged woman. Each

Barbara Dooling

day the cancer seems to smuggle some other part of me.

It is easy to have fear in the face of cancer. Living with what statistics say is a terminal illness is one grand task. The cancer has stolen a lot, but it has not robbed me of my spirit. And it cannot take away my hope. I am the one who dictates that! I shall not let it sweep. Perhaps this is the best thing that my husband sees in me. Yes, I believe this is the beauty that shines within me.

I undress in front of the mirror and allow myself to look at my imperfect body. I stare at the naked reflection. I search and do find my own beauty. I am petite. My muscle tone is still firm for the onset of my middle age. Though I am small breasted, I am well proportioned. The scar on my breast from the cancer is there but it is small and neatly concealed by a surgeon's skilled care. My stomach is flat and reveals no stretch marks. My face has smooth skin with high cheekbones. Despite my alopecia, loss of hair and eyelashes, my eyes are large, round, and prominent. They are such a deep, chocolate brown. They are dark and almost as black as an onyx gemstone. And they still shine!

I draw myself a warm bath, step into the tub slowly, and delicately lather my slender legs. The second scar on my body is on my thigh and rises to my hip. It too, is neat, although it is still purple from the newness of the surgical incision. I think to myself it's not so bad looking. I accept those imperfections. I find my own beauty. Tom takes my hand and gently lifts me out of the sudsy water. He kisses that scar on my breast as he has done many times over the years. It is as though he caresses and regards the old wound as something he himself has healed. He takes great care of my entire body. I do feel beautiful when I am in his arms—my love. He has stoked a fire inside of me that also cannot die. We have refused to allow the cancer to pirate away our intimacy. We retreat to our bed and make love.

When I grow weary of the beatings from the cancer and its treatments, Tom need only enter into my view, and I am renewed. My ardent lust for him is sparked! Chemo may snuff my appetite, but not my hunger for strong sexual desire. Our passion continues its boundless enthusiasm! We have taken full care of our marriage by nourishing it with all substances necessary to grow. Making love and the sensual side is just one portion—one single component. Our loyalty and laughter is another, and there is so much more. I appreciate his good humor. Indulging in laughter is an excellent way to fight pain. Tom has managed to make me chuckle during some extreme situations. Although I wasn't laughing when he shaved his head to match my bald noggin! Our Kara has his funny personality. Together they are such characters! I am so lucky to have them in my life. I refuse to dwell on my losses because it will only cloud my vision of all my many blessings.

March 23, 2002

Today marks the two year anniversary of a diagnosis of metastatic breast cancer. Truly, I am amazed that I am still here! And not only am I just here existing, I am thriving, living a beautiful life. Each breath is pure bliss. Tom and I are planning a vacation to Marco Island with our Kara-Girl. Not only will I be able to swim in the warm gulf, but I shall chase waves with Kara! I can even run after her! Yes, I've gained strength back in my leg, the one with all the new parts. My hip and femur are good and strong. At last I am able to endure long walks and even dancing! Lord, how I had missed dancing! Perhaps the most wonderful part of feeling healthy and well is playing with my girlie-girl again.

She is special! I hear her making wishes, and she always hopes

Barbara Dooling

for the same thing! No matter if it's on the first evening star, entering a new church, or a wish as she puffs out her birthday candles, she continues to wish for Mommy to get better. I tell her, "Kara, you can dream up a puppy, a castle, choose the biggest toy! You don't have to use all your wishes on me!" And my sweet child answers me, "Oh, but Mommy, you are the one I want the most. I don't like the cancer because it never seems to go away. I have to make you better—I just have to."

Tom's cousin Kevin has a fifteen year old son who is handicapped. Dana is a gift from God who has taught us plenty about love! During the past month, Dana underwent two ten hour surgeries at Children's Hospital to straighten his spine. Needless to say, not only did he need the great skill of the doctors and nurses, but he needed our prayers! Tom, Kara, and I visited Dana after the first surgery. When we entered the huge lobby of Children's Hospital, Kara pestered Tom for a penny to throw in the wishing pond in the lobby. We crowded around the other people, standing and looking at the fountain and all the shiny coins at the bottom. Kara tossed her copper cent, proposed a silent wish, and we were off to the elevators to visit her cousin. We didn't stay too long, as Dana was sleepy. Kara snuck her little arm up from the foot of his bed and signed him an "I love you" with her fingers. On our ride home, Kara seemed to have something on her mind. She never sits quietly in the back seat. She is usually full of chatter. In a soft, troublesome voice she said, "Mommy, I have something to tell you. It's a bad thing that I did." I could only imagine that she was fessing up to swiping something out of Dana's room or perhaps she wrote on the hospital wall with one of his crayons...

And what was the "bad thing" Kara had wished for when she plunked that penny into the wishing well? Dana to get better

Impossible Choices

instead of Mommy. I tried with all my might not to cry, but I did. And I explained to Kara that she was such a wonderful girl to make that very important wish. I told her that she could have wished for both Dana and me to be well. Better yet, I said that next time she can ask Daddy for another coin and make more wishes. Oh, my poor little Kara. I know how much she needs her mommy!

Kara has sacrificed plenty of time with me when I am hooked up to chemo, or at the doctor's or having some test. Even writing my book has taken precious moments away from us. How do I explain to her that the book is for her? She will often beckon to me to play house as I am furiously clicking away trying not to miss a deadline for the book. Kara might sneak her way into the spare room where I sit at the computer and tug on my sweater! I reach down and kiss her tiny nose, and tell her that even though Mommy can't be with her at that very moment, I am still with her in her heart, and that my spirit hovers over her. When she skins her knee at kindergarten, Mommy is with her there too. I told Kara to feel my warmth on her cheeks as tears trickle down. That's where Mommy is! I'll send her butterflies to chase and lady bugs to hold.

When I drop Kara off at school, I whisper to her that Mommy has a spirit which floats around her all day long. That's right my sweet daughter, I'm the sunshine on your shoulders, the breeze that makes your hair tickle your face, I am with you always!

This is what I say to her daddy, too! They both need to know that I am never more than a thought away. Jenna Rose has taught me this. That I am there even if their thoughts are busy at work and play. Tom has had to share me with the cancer, and split up our time together throughout the last two years while I wrote *Impossible Choices* for Kara. I have encouraged him to feel my presence all around him. He need only peek out the window to see my favorite

Barbara Dooling

flowers that he and I planted the first summer we bought our home. As he prunes our lovely rose bushes, I will be the last rose of summer still fresh on the vine. I'll pester him in September as he tries to rake the autumn leaves… yes, I am the bee that buzzes around his head. I'll be trying to get your attention, Tom, so don't be swatting at me! Don't ya see, Darling… I'll always be with you. I'll send you a rainbow on your grayest day, I'll wink an "I love you" with the twinkling north star. I am the dazzling glow in our daughter's big brown eyes. Scoop her up and squeeze her tight, and you'll both have me through the night. Come daybreak… at dawn… I'll be singing with the sparrows before your first yawn. No matter where I am or where you are… I'll always be with you… not very far!

ALWAYS WITH YOU:
My love for you is the shiniest treasure,
Nothing compares nor can measure.
Although we may be in different places,
You'll have our family's smiling faces.
For if it is me you wish to find,
Just close your eyes and call me to mind.
Surely you will laugh and remember,
Days gone by… January to December.
You, my husband and my dear sweet child,
Will never be without my guide.
I will be there day to day,
Steady and constant like the wind and the tide.
Never will we be apart,
My spirit surrounds you; my home is your heart.

About the Author

Barbara Dooling was born and raised Massachusetts with her parents and five older siblings. Although her youth was not idyllic, the challenges brought many blessings… most significantly her strong bonds between her brothers and sister, and a passion for writing. She kept a private journal of those days and now shares various passages with her readers in the hopes of communicating how love and commitment became an unbreakable force in her life that now sustains her through all of her adult challenges. She learned how to give and receive love; she learned the meaning of true love… that love isn't real until it's been tested. It was this love that she held out for while waiting for the "right man." She has given tiny pieces of her heart by sharing what she's learned. Professionally, Barbara enjoyed a seventeen year career in the medical industry, helping people with their daily struggles. As a wife and mother, she's spreading her wings to lift and protect her own family. Cancer and tragedy have invaded her perfect world. But she will persevere because "I love and I am loved!"

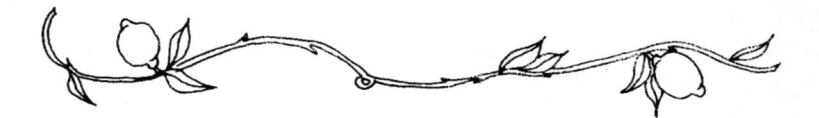

Other Novels by Huckleberry Press

www.HuckleberryPress.com

Dizzy Days

Gold Digger

The London File

Morning Star

Impossible Choices

A Time For Heroes

You Better Not Cry

Yummy